WHO'S PROTECTING THE PROTECTORS?

LEADERSHIP IN MENTAL HEALTH

GRANT EDWARDS

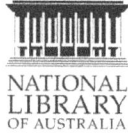

A catalogue record for this book is available from the National Library of Australia

NATIONAL LIBRARY OF AUSTRALIA

Publisher:
Inspiring Publishers
P.O. Box 159, Calwell, ACT Australia 2905
Email: inspiringpublisher.com
http://www.inspiringpublishers.com

National Library of Australia Cataloguing-in-Publication entry

Author: Grant Edwards

Title: **WHO'S PROTECTING THE PROTECTORS?**

ISBN: 978-1-922920-47-8 (Print)

✧

Chapter 1

Introduction

'Law enforcement officers are never "off duty".
They are dedicated public servants who are sworn to protect
public safety at any time and place that the peace is threatened.
They need all the help that they can get.'

— Barbara Boxer

L aw enforcement is not a career for everyone. It demands a special kind of individual, someone who can withstand the consistent and cumulative stresses of the job. These stresses affect not only the officers themselves but also their families, loved ones, and colleagues. Many who opt for a career in law enforcement view it as a calling, a desire to serve and protect others. But the toll of this profession can be high. Besides the array of physical injuries one might expect from a job that regularly involves violence, law enforcement officers are increasingly acknowledging the psychological impact of their work and the environments in which they operate. However, this calling to safeguard our society and community extracts a steep cost, both personal and professional, familial and financial.

When officers take their oath, they accept their responsibility to keep the public safe by protecting, serving, and enforcing laws. The training is thorough, rigorous, and specialised, covering areas such as the use of force, de-escalation techniques, cultural competency, and officer safety. The past 30 years have seen exponential advancements in technology, techniques, tradecraft, equipment, education, and training. Regrettably, the mental health of those who serve their communities hasn't been given the same level of attention.

Law enforcement agencies have invested millions in training and educating staff to ensure they are effective, efficient, and safe in their roles. Significant effort has also been dedicated to leadership development, equipping leaders to set the tone for their organisations and carry out the mission.

The success of any law enforcement agency critically depends on leadership. Leaders provide direction, guidance to their subordinates, and work to uphold morale. A leader must navigate the challenges of the job while guiding and directing the agency. Effective communication with both the agency's staff and the public is crucial, as is inspiring confidence in the agency's ability to protect the community. A leader must make tough decisions, often in life-or-death situations, and have the courage to stand for what is right, even when it is unpopular.

Respect and trust from both the agency's staff and the community are essential for a successful leader. This individual must be trustworthy and consistently act in the best interest of the agency and the people it serves.

Successful law enforcement leaders possess several positive traits, including integrity, empathy, trustworthiness, honesty, and respect for the law. Excellent communication skills, the ability to motivate their team, and the courage to make difficult decisions under stress are vital. Furthermore, a strong sense of justice and fairness, leading by example, and the willingness to learn from mistakes are also important. Any law enforcement leader aspiring to succeed in their role must strive for excellence in every aspect of their job, embodying these essential traits.

Regrettably, the emphasis, investment, and training on mental health, and the ways in which the job impacts it, have been insufficient.

A law enforcement leader with negative traits can be harmful to both the organisation and the community. These traits may include a lack of integrity, an inability to accept responsibility, a disregard for others, and poor team management skills. A leader displaying these traits might struggle with decision-making, effective communication, and handling difficult situations. Moreover, such a leader may find it challenging to build relationships with other law enforcement agencies or community members. Ultimately, these negative traits can undermine officer morale and erode trust in the department's leadership.

These behaviours can profoundly impact staff mental health. Leadership in mental health involves managing and guiding individuals, teams, and organisations to promote positive mental health outcomes. Leaders in this field must recognise and address the unique needs of those with mental health issues and advocate for their rights. They should foster an environment encouraging open dialogue, collaboration, and support. Furthermore, leaders must be aware of available resources for mental health issues and provide guidance on accessing them. Finally, they must comprehend the legal implications of mental health issues within the law enforcement context.

Law enforcement leaders play a crucial role in prioritising staff mental health. They should ensure that staff are aware of resources like mental health services and support networks and feel encouraged to seek help if needed. They must provide adequate training to help staff identify signs of mental distress in themselves and others, and to respond appropriately. By promoting an open culture within their organisation, leaders can make their staff feel comfortable discussing mental health issues and feel safe and supported in performing their duties.

The high-pressure nature of law enforcement, potential exposure to violence and danger, and organisational injustices can contribute to significant stress levels. This stress can trigger physical symptoms like headaches, fatigue, insomnia, and digestive problems, and psychological issues such as depression, anxiety, post-traumatic stress disorder (PTSD), and substance abuse. It can strain personal relationships and family life. Moreover, officers may experience traumatic events causing long-term mental health problems. It's crucial for law enforcement personnel to be trained to recognise and manage stress and mental health issues to maintain their and their colleagues' well-being.

The data is clear: law enforcement officers are up to four times more likely to suffer a mental health condition during their employment than the general public. They are also more likely to die up to 20 years earlier due to the effects of mental health and stress-related injuries.

After my personal experiences with post-traumatic stress, depression, and anxiety, I recognised a significant gap in mental health leadership within the law enforcement community. So, I began researching the subject more broadly. To my surprise, I found little information on the topic, especially within law enforcement. This gap was glaringly obvious.

Working alongside law enforcement agencies worldwide, it became clear to me that wellness and mental health in the workplace are critical issues. However, for many, the opportunity to discuss or acknowledge these topics is unavailable. Numerous reasons prevent law enforcement personnel from discussing their mental health.

This book aims to equip those in leadership roles with the knowledge and skills to move beyond awareness, filling the gap in mental health leadership. The goal is to develop and implement effective strategies and programs to support their teams and cultivate resilient, positive organisational mental health programs.

To provide context, I share my personal experience of suffering a mental illness, including my suicide attempt and discuss my journey towards better mental health, detailing how I gained understanding and skills to identify, support, and guide someone who is suffering. I explore the challenges that often prevent leaders and organisations from progressing a mental health program and discuss the elements of law enforcement culture that impede the successful uptake of support programs. I also share how I managed the grief and moral injury from not being able to support friends and colleagues who took their own lives.

Critically, I emphasise the importance of leaders taking care of their own mental health and share my strategies for doing so. I draw from a combination of my life experiences, my 34-year tenure with the Australian Federal Police (18 of those years as a senior executive), and my academic qualifications in leadership, policy, and governance. Finally, as an elite athlete and qualified coach, I share my health and wellbeing lessons.

I hope you find this book insightful. By using its content, I hope you can further your development, support your team, and potentially challenge your organisation to establish a meaningful, sustainable, and reliable mental health and wellbeing program.

Chapter 2

My Story

'I wasn't faking being sick; I was faking being well.'
– unknown

To provide context for this book, I feel it is important to outline my own mental health journey.

Between 1985 and 2019, I served as a police officer. I took pride in doing my utmost to keep my community and country safe from the insidious criminals who prey on Australia's good and innocent people. I witnessed and experienced the worst humanity had to offer and the lengths to which criminals would go to exploit, harm, and profit from their victims.

Never in my wildest dreams did I think I would become a mental health statistic. Not only was I diagnosed with post-traumatic stress, but I also became one of the many law enforcement officers worldwide who would attempt to take their own life.

I had always known that I would pursue a career in law enforcement. It was in my DNA. Like many who join the force, it was my life's purpose, and it became my identity. I wanted to make a difference for my family, my community, and my country.

My life changed forever on August 11, 1985. I found myself sitting in a room with other aspiring individuals, eager to begin my career in the Australian Federal Police (AFP). The excitement was palpable. I can still vividly recall the moment when a larger-than-life station sergeant walked into the room and announced, in a deep, gruff voice:

> *'Today, you lose your identity, you lose your name, you become a number – the number we assign to you as an Australian Federal Police Officer... If you don't like that... well, get up and leave now.'*

I thought, wow, this is the real deal! A number of people stood straight up and opted to leave, but many of us stayed.

From the time I entered the academy, I was subjected to an overwhelming amount of information designed to shape me into the best law enforcement officer possible. They brought me to the peak of physical fitness, put me through a series of physical tests, and educated me about the law and how to enforce it. I was drilled on organisational procedures, governance, and protocols that I was expected to adhere to. I spent countless hours learning and practicing self-defence to ensure my safety. Weekly, they instructed me on the use of force techniques, how to de-escalate potentially violent situations, and the effective use of handcuffs, batons, and OC spray. Importantly, a considerable amount of time was devoted to training me in the execution of lethal force. I had become adept at maintaining emotional neutrality and was taught how to remain impassive in difficult and critical situations. They shaped me to distrust and question everything, never to take any answer, event, or situation at face value. This led to a deep-seated distrust that permeated all aspects of my life.

One element that was never mentioned, let alone taught, was the potential for being psychologically affected by the work we would eventually undertake, and how I could better prepare myself and manage the impacts of the job I was about to embark upon.

I had an inherent understanding that 'the job' was tough. I had two uncles in the NSW Police Force, and I saw how their roles affected their health. But we never spoke about it; we just acknowledged it and moved on. I knew it could be a demanding career, yet my early training did not prepare me for the traumatic and tragic experiences that come with being a law enforcement officer.

In my early days, work was intense. I regularly worked long hours, sometimes more than 24 straight, to the point of absolute exhaustion. Shift work resulted in unhealthy sleep habits, altered my eating patterns, and led me to stop exercising. I spent disproportionate amounts of time away from home due to last-minute assignments, missing holidays and many crucial events like my children's birthdays and milestone celebrations. Over the years, my stress and anxiety levels insidiously crept higher and higher, a change to which I was oblivious.

Throughout my career, I endured verbal abuse, physical assaults, spitting, biting, and being targeted with urine and faeces. I suffered cuts, abrasions, sprains, and broken bones. I dealt with horrendous crimes, homicides, rapes, assaults, and fatal motor vehicle accidents. I saw humans beheaded, children exposed to the horrific impacts of chemical weapons. I removed infants suffering from welts, bruises, and sores from flea-infested, maggot-ridden homes. I encountered children, some as young as six months old, horrifically abused, sexually assaulted, and molested to satisfy the inhuman desires of some individuals.

I would find myself in hospital operating theatres with doctors trying to save the life of drug traffickers who attempted to internally import drugs over the border. I would deal with a drug overdose victim whose 'friends' were so high they used the chord of an iron to try and electrically jump-start his heart after he had died.

'... I've seen some bad things... I come from a warrior culture.... and I am not supposed to be affected by my job... but I was... and couldn't tell anyone in my agency... lest I would be considered weak...'

During my service, I was deployed to hostile countries where I was forcefully removed from a vehicle at gunpoint by the local military and attacked by Taliban insurgents in Kabul who detonated their bomb vests and indiscriminately shot at anything that moved. I contracted life-threatening diseases like tick paralysis, chikungunya, dengue fever, and schistosomiasis, which have left me with lifelong debilitating consequences.

While giving evidence in court, my integrity, professionalism, and credibility were frequently attacked by defence lawyers who had never left the comfort and sanctity of school, university, or their plush offices. I was often ridiculed, patronised, and mocked in front of my peers, the jury, and judiciary, without the opportunity to defend myself. Worst of all, criminals attempted to physically and psychologically threaten and intimidate both me and my family.

At times, I faced bullying, threats, and derision from peers and superiors. I chose to focus on my physical health outside of work and seldom participated in social events. In my early days, the culture deemed it more acceptable to indulge in a lengthy lunch or alcohol than to work towards fitness and health. This was just how things were, and I accepted that.

It was 2013, and I had just returned from a 12-month deployment to Afghanistan, resuming my role as the AFP aviation commander in Queensland. This role made me responsible for the aviation security component of the G20 conference in Brisbane.

Despite my experiences, I never anticipated becoming a mental health statistic. In late 2013, after my return from Afghanistan, I began experiencing physical and psychological problems. The best way to describe it was feeling 'odd' or sensing that 'things were not right.' I became increasingly tense, impatient, irritable, intolerant, sad, and angry. Even the most minor noise caused me to startle. I had become hyper-vigilant, unnaturally alert to potential dangers, whether real or imagined. I couldn't control my thoughts or reactions. My mind became a muddle of confusing thoughts, impairing my ability to think logically and coherently. I had become a prisoner in my own mind, with no means of escape. I avoided friends, colleagues, and family, effectively becoming a recluse. Debilitating migraines, muscle and joint aches, and constant stomach churn immobilised me. Sleep had become a source of fear due to intrusive dreams that seemed to play on an endless loop, causing fatigue to consume my waking hours. In a futile attempt to relax and sleep, I turned to alcohol and over-the-counter drugs, teetering on the brink of addiction. My brain had convinced me that I had become a burden to my family, friends, and colleagues. I had lost my identity, my drive, my commitment, and my love for life.

My mind couldn't reconcile what was happening to me. After all, I was the tough, stoic cop, impervious to everything. I was the fit and healthy former elite athlete who had represented his country in five different sports and played American football at the University of Hawaii. I was the strongman who could pull trucks, buses, trams, airplanes, sailing ships, locomotive trains, and huge mining trucks.

As my health continued to decline, I felt increasingly out of control. In my mind, I had become a burden to my family and loved ones, an imposition to my colleagues and friends, and an embarrassment to myself. It seemed as if everything I had worked for throughout my life had become worthless, mirroring how I felt about myself.

I'll never forget 'the day.' That's what I call it. It was the day my life came to a standstill, the day I attempted to take my own life. I was driving to work in the early morning winter dimness just before dawn, en route to another day of endless meetings on security arrangements for the 2014 G20 Summit. The physical and psychological pain I was enduring was at its peak. In the preceding weeks, I had contemplated and ideated suicide. Things seemed so dark. Although I could hardly think straight, moments of clarity would surface when I contemplated suicide. It was an odd sensation. I can't explain why I could meticulously plan multiple scenarios for ending my life, yet I couldn't carry out basic cognitive activities outside this realm of clarity.

On this particular morning, my thoughts escalated to a point where the only option I saw was to end my pain and leave this world. I attempted to take my own life, and in doing so, I became a statistic.

Eventually, I was diagnosed with complex post-traumatic stress injury (PTSI) and high-functioning unipolar depression. I believed this diagnosis would end my career, bring me embarrassment, cause my family shame, and leave my future uncertain.

The subsequent years saw me embark on a lifelong journey of self-reflection and intensive therapy sessions with psychiatrists, psychologists, psychotherapists, medical specialists, dietitians, nutritionists, physiotherapists, massage therapists, and integrative medical practitioners.

My journey to improved mental health continues today. It's not a linear process but a rather complex one. I never thought I was suffering from a mental health issue. I was referred to several medical specialists to understand why I was feeling and behaving the way I was. I underwent a plethora of tests, being poked and prodded beyond belief.

✦

Chapter 3

What Is Mental Illness?

'Mental illness is like fighting a war where the enemy's strategy is to convince you that a war isn't actually happening.'

— unknown

Mental health, as the foundation for individuals' well-being and effective functioning, extends beyond the absence of a mental disorder. It involves our ability to think, learn, understand our emotions, and the reactions of others. Mental health is a state of balance, both externally and internally. It encompasses a range of experiences and situations, from mental wellbeing through to severe and enduring mental illnesses affecting a person's overall emotional and psychological condition. Life events such as bereavement, financial difficulties, and personal happiness can lead to depression and anxiety.

Mental health includes emotional, psychological, and social well-being. It influences cognition, perception, and behaviour. It also determines how an individual handles stress, interpersonal relationships, and decision-making. Mental health may include an individual's ability to enjoy life and create a balance between life activities and efforts to achieve psychological resilience. Cultural differences, subjective assessments, and competing professional theories all affect how one defines 'mental health.' Some early signs of mental health problems include sleep disturbances, lack of energy, and thoughts of self-harm or harming others.

Yet, Mental health problems are a significant public health concern worldwide. In most developed nations, these issues are the leading cause of disability and contribute substantially to the overall burden of disease. Mental health problems correlate with several negative outcomes, including poor physical health, reduced life expectancy, unemployment, and poverty.

According to the World Health Organization, mental health disorders are the leading cause of disability globally[1]. In 2017, an estimated 300 million people were living with depression, and 260 million were grappling with anxiety disorders. Alarmingly, suicide is now the second leading cause of death among individuals aged 15 – 29.

Many less developed nations lack adequate access to mental health services and support for those in desperate need. Unfortunately, their problems often go undiagnosed and untreated.

The prevalence of mental health problems is increasing. In developed nations, the incidence of mental illness has surged by nearly 50% over the past two decades. This rise is due, in part, to increasing awareness of mental health problems and the availability of improved treatments[2].

The understanding and treatment of mental illness have evolved significantly over the centuries. The earliest theories often attributed the peculiar symptoms of mental illness to supernatural forces like demonic possession, sorcery, curses, or an angry deity. This perspective experienced a radical shift around 400 BC when the Greek physician Hippocrates began to view mental illness as a physiological ailment, rather than a

1   https://www.who.int/news-room/fact-sheets/detail/mental-disorders
2   https://www.nimh.nih.gov/health/statistics/mental-illness

'...Mental health is not talked about in my agency... I had a female officer who worked for me... She had just had a miscarriage... I could see she was suffering but had no idea how to help her. My boss was a command-and-control leader... he pushed and pushed her to do things because she was so good at her work... She came to me in tears and talked about wanting to take her life as the pressure was too much... I did what I could and it helped, but I had never been taught on how to take care of my staff as a leader...'

result of demonic influences or divine displeasure. By the 8th century, Muslim Arabs established the first asylums to house the mentally ill.

Mental illness has historically been a burden to both the affected individual and their family. Those suffering from mental health problems were frequently stigmatised and mistreated. Families often concealed their mentally ill relatives, confining them to a single room to prevent exposure to society. In other instances, mentally ill individuals were abandoned in standard hospitals without proper attention or care. Tragically, those with no family or whose families rejected them were left to perish on the streets[3].

These attitudes contributed to the stigma, shame, and discrimination associated with mental health problems, which continue to pervade our society today. Derogatory terms like 'nutter,' 'crazy,' and 'madman' are often used to label individuals with mental health conditions. Such statements, rich in stigma and negativity, can be deeply harmful, often exacerbating the struggle that many face in seeking acknowledgment and help.

---

3   https://www.healthyplace.com/other-info/mental-illness-overview/the-history-of-mental-illness

Reflecting the growing global concern, in 2021, the United Nations General Assembly dedicated its World Health Organization's (WHO) forum to mental health for the first time, emphasizing the urgent need to prioritize mental health and stimulate new investment in this critical area[4].

Here are a few numbers that are confronting and validate this need:

- Mental health has quickly become one of the most talked about topics across society. Make no mistake, the greatest cause of disability globally is poor mental health and in the workplace it's an urgent priority. Mental disorders are on the rise and will cost the global economy $16 trillion (USD) by 2030[5] with about 12 billion working days lost every year[6].
- The mortality rate of those with mental disorders is significantly higher than the general population, with a median life expectancy loss of 10.1 years.
- It is estimated that mental disorders are attributable to 14.3% of deaths worldwide, or approximately 8 million deaths each year.

Yet, mental health problems are treatable. With appropriate treatment, most people with mental health problems can recover and lead productive lives.

---

4   https://www.who.int/campaigns/world-mental-health-day/2021/about#:~: text=During%20the%20World%20Health%20Assembly%20in%20May%20 2021%2C,updated%20implementation%20options%20and%20indicators%20for%20 measuring%20progress.

5   The Lancet Commission on global mental health and sustainable development (2018). The Lancet, Vol. 392, No. 10157. (October 10).

6   LaMontagne, A. D., Martin, A., Page, K. M., Reavley, N. J., Noblet, A. J., Milner, A. J., et al. (2014). Workplace mental health: developing an integrated intervention approach. BMC Psychiatry, 14(1), 131.

✧

Chapter 4

The Mental Health Problem In Law Enforcement

'Law enforcement is in the midst of a mental health crisis.'
– James Comey, former director of the Federal Bureau
of Investigation (FBI), and retired New York City and
Los Angeles Police Department Commissioner
— William J. Bratton

Throughout my law enforcement career, I seldom considered the significant impact this job had on the mental health of those in the service. While I acknowledged that being a law enforcement officer was stressful, I didn't truly understand the mental toll it could take until I delved into leadership and mental health. My research revealed that law enforcement officers are at a heightened risk of developing mental health issues, such as depression and post-traumatic stress disorder, due to frequent exposure to traumatic events and high-stress situations. This realisation underscored the importance of leaders in law enforcement recognising and prioritising the mental health of their officers. Leaders must provide support and resources to ensure their officers can manage both the physical and psychological demands of their jobs.

It's well-known that the mental health of law enforcement officers has long been neglected by the profession and its organisations. For centuries, it was a taboo subject. Current statistics continue to confirm this, presenting a grim picture of the state of mental health among those who have sworn to protect and serve their communities.

Law enforcement work is stressful, dangerous, and complex. Officers frequently encounter the worst aspects of humanity and must make split-second life-or-death decisions, all while operating within slim margins for error. The profession is psychologically taxing and physically draining.

Thankfully, the recent rise in law enforcement suicides has spurred conversation and awareness around this topic, hoping to curb this alarming trend. Many law enforcement departments worldwide have established mental health programs to protect their officers' mental health proactively. These programs have proved beneficial for many officers. Yet, there are still barriers to progress, misunderstandings, and lack of clarity about what a comprehensive wellness and mental health program should entail.

Regrettably, leadership in mental health within these departments has often been neglected. Many leaders have not been educated or trained in mental health leadership because there are scant programs, tools, and training in this area. Many leaders grapple with recognizing and addressing staff members suffering from mental health issues. This is entirely understandable, as confronting mental health in the workplace can be a complex challenge. The rapid rise in workplace mental health issues poses difficulties not only in managing the repercussions but also in implementing preventative measures.

Many individuals in law enforcement find themselves overwhelmed and immobilized by the enormity of the mental health issues facing their profession. The stigma surrounding mental health and the suicide epidemic are pressing issues. However, it's high time we bridged the gap between comprehension and concrete action. This situation necessitates recognising the vital role of leadership in addressing these issues.

By the time I was plunged into the grim task of investigating child exploitation and sex trafficking, I had already earned my detective qualifications and completed the requisite education and training in leadership for my designation.

> *'...I was suffering with PTSI and tried to talk to my senior boss about what I was going through... he just listened, but he seemed distracted and not interested... He shook my hand and said that he hoped I feel better soon!... His poor response nearly destroyed me...'*

Though mental health was a crucial concern, there was no reference to, acknowledgement of, or training offered on it, let alone any leadership training on the subject. My small team of five, myself included, triaged allegations of Australians accessing child exploitation material. In the early days, many of the referrals were related to material being exchanged through the post. However, with the growing availability of the internet, we saw a rapid increase in material being accessed and exchanged via computers. At its worst in 2003, we were receiving about 9,000 referrals of Australians attempting to access child exploitation material online. Our role was to examine each of these referrals to determine the level of criminality, but our priority was to identify any child at immediate risk of physical harm. During these early years, there was no requirement for psychological assessments, nor were there any psychological support services provided to us.

Back then, I was aware that the stress and trauma associated with this type of crime presented external challenges to the team's wellness. However, I was not cognisant that my team could be vulnerable to experiencing compassion fatigue, moral injury, and burnout. Compassion fatigue, which results from empathising with the suffering children, is associated with feelings of anger, anxiety, guilt, hopelessness, and powerlessness. Additional symptoms may include emotional instability, diminished self-esteem, self-harm, inability to concentrate, hypervigilance, disorientation, rigidity, apathy, perfectionism, and preoccupation with trauma. The mere involvement in investigating child exploitation could induce a moral injury, as officers witness or partake in acts that contradict their deeply held moral beliefs. The negative health outcomes, as I would learn, could include the risk of sleep disorders, cardiovascular disease, reliance on alcohol and over-the-counter medications as coping mechanisms, posttraumatic stress disorder, and suicide. Unfortunately, I would see many of my team members succumb to most of these outcomes.

Having been unable to secure any formal psychological support from my organisation, I took it upon myself to reach out to one of the new psychologists that had recently joined us. This individual agreed to meet with my team to discuss strategies for managing the stressors we were grappling with. Despite my uncertainty about how to orchestrate such a meeting and what to anticipate, I arranged a gathering in a neutral, comfortable environment. We spent a day there, talking amongst ourselves about our work. At the end of this day, after the psychologist had left, I was keen to know how the team felt about the experience. To my surprise, when I posed the question, their collective response was overwhelmingly positive. Each person declared that they felt significantly better after the day's events.

This positive feedback initially buoyed me, but I was soon brought back to earth when I pressed for details. They admitted that their improved morale stemmed from the fact that the psychologist had spent much of the time discussing his own struggles. According to them, this made them feel much better about their own situations. Though this was not the outcome I had anticipated, it did indicate that we had started a conversation about mental health, and I viewed that as a step in the right direction.

What has become clear to me is that we are collectively failing our first responders and their families across the globe when it comes to mental health. Whether I'm watching the news, scrolling through social media or hearing anecdotes from serving members about how the operational landscape has notably deteriorated, I am confronted by numerous stories of chaos, stress, violence, uncertainty, and stigma occupying their minds.

Chapter 5
Stressors of the Job

*'Officers wear protective clothing and other equipment
to keep themselves safe from physical harm. However,
there isn't any protective equipment that can keep them safe
from the psychological damage many face.'*

— Unknown

The effects of stressors on law enforcement personnel can be widespread and detrimental. These stressors can precipitate physical, mental, and emotional exhaustion, resulting in reduced job performance and an escalation in burnout. Consequently, morale among officers may diminish, undermining their effectiveness in fulfilling their duties. Moreover, these stressors can trigger higher rates of absenteeism and turnover among officers, culminating in a loss of productivity and efficiency within the department.

Stressors can also adversely affect relationships — those between officers and their families or friends, as well as those between officers and the public they serve. Stress conditions can further inhibit their ability to carry out their duties effectively[7]:

---

7   Dane Subošić, Slaviša Krstić, and Ivana Luknar, 'Police Subculture and Potential Stress Risks,' (paper, *Security Concepts and Policies New Generation Conference*, Ohrid, MK, July 2018).

- **External stressors** – Jurisdictional isolation, seemingly ineffective legal and court systems, adverse media accounts, impact of negative and venomous social media
- **Internal stressors** – Poor supervision and leadership, absence of career development opportunities, inadequate reward system, unpleasant policies, over-reporting, mountains of paperwork and budgetary constraints
- **Performance stressors** – Role ambiguity and conflict, adverse work and roster schedules, inherent fear and danger, sense of uselessness, and absence of closure
- **Individual stressors** – Feeling overcome by fear and danger, pressures to conform, gender disparity, bullying, sexual harassment, ethnicity and cultural differences, lack of unique understanding of such demographics as the LGBQTI community
- **Life-threatening stressors** – Ever-present potential for injury or death to the individual, fellow law enforcement, or members of the public
- **Social isolation stressors** – Cynicism, isolation, and alienation from the community; prejudice and discrimination
- **Organisational stressors** – Administrative philosophy, changing of policies and procedures, morale, job satisfaction, and misdirected performance measures
- **Functional stressors** – Role conflict/confusion, use of discretion, and legal mandates/obligations
- **Personal stressors** – Home life, including personal issues, spousal, illness, problems with children and aging parents, marital distress, and financial constraints
- **Physiological stressors** – Fatigue, medical conditions, comorbid health issues, poor sleep, poor nutrition
- **Psychological stressors** – All the above and the exposure to shocking situations

'...I'd seen, smelt, and heard many horrible things over my career... my senses were overwhelmed.. rather than help me, my department pensioned me out.. I was left to fend for myself..I felt alone, a pariah, a failure..'

Two recent studies reveal the impact poor mental health has on law enforcement officers. A 2017 study conducted by researchers at the University of Toronto, Canada[8] demonstrated the dangers of failing to acknowledge and deal with mental health among police. Researchers' interviews found that first responders with mental health injuries exhibited 'performance deficits on complex cognitive tasks', which could include tasks that required first responders to assess risks, plan multi-step responses to an emergency, especially complex operations where there are multiple offenders and/or victims. The risk to society is high if these health issues are not dealt with appropriately.

A 2018 Cambridge University study of police in the UK revealed two-thirds of all respondents said they had a mental health issue directly resulting from police work. Yet almost all the survey's respondents — some 93% — said they would go to work as usual if suffering from psychological issues such as stress or depression. They would do so without seeking treatment because of the associated negative organisational stress and affects[9].

---

8   Regehr, C., & LeBlanc, V.R. (2017). 'PTSD, acute stress, performance and decision-making in emergency service workers.' *Journal of the American Academy of Psychiatry and the Law,* 45(2), 184-192. doi: 10.1037/t12199-000

9   Hargreaves, J., Husband, H., & Linehan, C. (2018). Police workforce, England and Wales, 31 March 2018. *Statistical Bulletin,* 11(18).

Law enforcement officers are often expected to display exceptional strength in dangerous situations, standing as stalwart protectors of their communities and displaying the courage to run towards danger when others are fleeing from it. However, their minds and bodies bear the scars of a continuous exposure to trauma, stressful events, and organisational injustices, eventually reaching a tipping point where their resilience wanes. Despite their steadfast commitment to their occupational responsibilities, it's crucial to remember that they are humans, not invincible.

Disturbingly, within law enforcement, almost one in four officers has contemplated suicide. More officers die by suicide than by homicide — in fact, the rate is 2.3 times higher. Their mental deterioration is often dismissed as a regrettable but unavoidable aspect of their work. Law enforcement work is not only stressful and dangerous, but also frequently stigmatised. Officers must make split-second life-and-death decisions, with slim and unforgiving margins for error.

Adding insult to injury, many police officers face a culture of silence and disregard for mental health challenges. While they are trained to interact with people suffering from mental illnesses, many officers are not given the care and attention they need to cope with their own traumas.

The evidence suggests that many in law enforcement will experience a mental health injury during their career, and most within the profession will know someone who has suffered similarly. Today, law enforcement personnel are nine times more likely to succumb to psychological stress-related injuries, have a reduced life expectancy due to constant exposure to traumatic events, and are three times more likely to experience relationship and divorce issues. Yet, the majority must battle hostile workplaces and insurance agencies for extended periods to secure treatment[10], law enforcement officers report much higher rates of depression, burnout, post-traumatic stress injury (PTSI), and anxiety than the general population.

Many develop maladaptive behaviours like a reliance on alcohol and non-prescription drugs, self-isolation, sleeping too much, lashing out at others, spending excessive amounts of time alone, not participating in activities that were once enjoyed, avoidance of social situations, and loss of interest in previously engaging activities.

---

10 https://www.waldenu.edu/programs/criminal-justice/resource/five-reasons-the-mental-health-of-police-officers-needs-to-be-a-priority#:~:text=According%20 to%20the%20latest%20law%20enforcement%20statistics%20by,at%20least%20 once%20in%20their%20lifetime.%201%202.

✧

Chapter 6

Burnout – It's A Real Problem

'Mastering others is strength. Mastering yourself is true power.'
— Lao Tzu, Taoist philosopher

When I speak with people within law enforcement and ask, 'What are you doing for your health and wellbeing?' I consistently hear, 'I just can't find time in the day' to commit to a regime. Most of us can't find time, so you have to create it and then commit to using that time for self-maintenance.

More than ever, our lives are swamped with the expectation to do more in the workplace. Sure, we hear the mantra urging us to seek a healthier balance between our work and personal lives, yet many seldom achieve such equilibrium, leading to increased stress.

The stress of everyday life is problematic enough, but when combined with our busy personal lives and work commitments, we can become overwhelmed. For many in law enforcement, you may recognise the extreme level of stress you're experiencing in your life, but you might not immediately identify your situation. More than likely, it's burnout.

Burnout is recognised as a state of emotional, mental, and often physical exhaustion brought on by prolonged or repeated stress. While it's most often caused by problems at work, it can also occur in other life areas, such as parenting, caregiving, or romantic relationships.

Burnout isn't simply a result of working long hours or juggling too many tasks, although both contribute. The cynicism, depression, and lethargy characteristic of burnout most often occur when a person is burdened by unreasonable workplace expectations.

Burnout can manifest itself in physical symptoms and emotional and behavioural symptoms, including headaches, fatigue, heartburn, and other gastrointestinal issues, poor sleep, as well as increased potential for alcohol, drug, or food misuse. Most people at one time during their law enforcement career would feel burnt out and experience exhaustion.

Burnout in the law enforcement workplace is a real and pressing issue. It's a state of physical, emotional, and mental exhaustion brought on by excessive and long-lasting stress. Various factors can contribute to it, including lengthy hours, heavy workloads, lack of control over one's work, and lack of job satisfaction.

When I pledged to become a law enforcement officer, I took an oath of service to protect and assist my community. I committed to prioritising service over self; an honourable intention, yet it was the start of a downward spiral into poor mental health.

As a newly commissioned officer freshly graduated from the academy, I was in the best physical shape of my life. I'd passed a series of physical and psychological assessments, proving my mental health was in good shape. Tragically, over the course of my career, I experienced physical illness and emotional suffering with devastating consequences. Yet I knew nothing else but to pick myself up, lock away the problems, and continue doing what I loved.

The job rarely afforded me the time and space to deal with the continually mounting stress. I had no time to decompress, reflect, and understand the job's effects on me. Even though I tried to maintain my physical fitness, the job always took precedence. I had never considered caring for my mental health.

If we don't make efforts to care for ourselves and continue to neglect our mind, body, and soul, we're destined for a life of poor health. It's not unreasonable to dedicate one hour a day to self-care. One hour equates to 1/24 of your day, less than 5%.

Psychologists Herbert Freudenberger and Gail North developed a 12-stage model of burnout that affects so many leaders today[11]. Here's what to look out for:

> '...It's hard to go to sleep each night... my mind plays a continuous reel of the things I've seen and been exposed to over the years... now I find I'm too scared to close my eyes... how do you unsee what you've seen? You can't....'

Stage 1: Excessive ambition

While ambition is a positive trait that supports our personal and professional goals, it can quickly become detrimental when excessive. Excessive ambition often arises when you feel the need to prove yourself – whether to yourself or to others.

Stage 2: Working harder

You establish work-focused primary goals, relegating all other aspects of your life to secondary importance.

Stage 3: Neglecting personal needs

When your personal needs are sacrificed – such as not having time to exercise, cook nutritious meals, or maintain regular sleep hygiene – the effects manifest. These include unhealthy weight gain, insomnia, decreased focus, brain fog, and lack of drive.

Stage 4: Displacement of conflicts and needs

Due to an excessive focus on work, problems are often dismissed or left unaddressed, leading to feelings of threat, panic, and jitteriness.

Stage 5: No longer any need for non-work-related needs

Friends, family, and self-care are often dismissed as being irrelevant or not as important.

Stage 6: Increasing denial of the problem

In this stage, you may perceive your collaborators or co-workers as undisciplined or lazy. Excuses are often made, suggesting that problems are solely caused by time pressure and work, rather than any life changes. The phrase *'If only I had more time, then...'* is common, indicating a sense of detachment from reality.

Stage 7: Withdrawal, lack of direction, cynicism

Similar to stage 5, there is little to no room for a social life, and often, there's a need to relieve stress using alcohol or drugs.

Stage 8: Behavioural changes/psychological reactions

Changes in behaviour are unique to each individual, but family and friends may notice discernible alterations in demeanour and conduct.

Stage 9: Depersonalisation: loss of contact with self and personal needs

At this point, you're unable to recognise your own value. The drive that once propelled you diminishes, and you may contemplate quitting, moving, or making a significant life decision.

Stage 10: Inner emptiness, anxiety, addictive behaviour

Lack of enthusiasm or interest in work leads to destructive behaviour, potentially including excessive alcohol and drug use. Activities are often exaggerated.

Stage 11: Increasing feeling of meaninglessness and lack of interest

Feelings of being lost, exhausted, anxious, and hopeless about your life, your mission, and your values become prevalent.

Stage 12: Physical exhaustion that can be life-threatening

This stage can include a total mental and physical collapse, necessitating immediate medical attention.

The benefits of avoiding burnout in the workplace are numerous. Firstly, it can help to reduce absenteeism and presenteeism, which can negatively affect productivity. Secondly, it can lead to improved morale among employees, as they feel more supported in their work environment. Finally, it can contribute to enhancing job satisfaction and employee engagement, leading to increased productivity and overall better performance.

✧

Chapter 7

Barriers To Help-Seeking Behaviour

'Mental illness is nothing to be ashamed of,
but stigma and bias shame us all.'
— Former US President Bill Clinton

The question I am most often asked within law enforcement is: *'Why don't people get help?'* The ubiquitous response is *'the stigma'*. The reasons, however, are far broader and more complex than that.

It's universally recognised that impediments to help-seeking can have negative ramifications for individuals, families, and organisations. Help-seeking is a multifaceted behaviour, influenced by an array of personal, social, and environmental factors. Consequently, obstacles to help-seeking can be perceived as multi-dimensional, with distinct barriers functioning at different levels.

At the individual level, personal factors such as shame, embarrassment, fear of stigma, and a lack of knowledge about services and resources can all influence help-seeking behaviour. Social elements, including family dynamics, peer pressure, and community norms, can also steer an individual's decision to seek help.

Contextual factors, such as poverty, discrimination, and structural violence, can additionally construct barriers to help-seeking.

At the family level, obstacles to help-seeking can include a lack of familial support, communication difficulties, and a dearth of knowledge about services and resources.

At the organisational level, barriers to help-seeking can include inadequate support, a lack of knowledge about services and resources, and a deficit of trust in service providers.

Specific to law enforcement, some barriers are:

Stigma

Mental health stigma refers to societal disapproval, or when society shames people living with a mental illness or seeking help for emotional distress. The pressure of mental health stigma can emanate from family, friends, co-workers, and broader society. Groups can also politicise stigma . It can inhibit people living with mental illness from getting help, integrating into society, and leading fulfilling lives.

Stigma is a negative and often unjust social attitude assigned to a person or group, frequently attributing shame to them for a perceived deficiency or difference in their existence. Individuals or groups can apply stigma to those who live a certain way, possess certain cultural beliefs or lifestyle choices, or to people living with health conditions, such as mental illnesses.

Mental health stigma can stem from stereotypes—simplified or generalised beliefs or depictions of entire groups of people that are often inaccurate, negative, and offensive. They facilitate quick judgments about others based on a few defining characteristics, which are then applied to anyone in that group. For instance, people living with depression are often unjustly characterised as 'lazy', while those with anxiety may be labelled 'cowardly'. Many people fear being deemed 'crazy' merely for seeking support from a therapist. These characterisations are neither valid nor informed, often leading to pain and preventing people from seeking the help they need[12].

Stigma arises from a lack of understanding of mental illness (due to ignorance and misinformation), and because some people harbour negative attitudes or beliefs towards it (prejudice). This can result in discrimination against people with mental illness.

Stigma can incite discrimination. Discrimination can be overt and direct, such as someone making a derogatory remark about your mental illness or your treatment. Alternatively, it might be unintentional or subtle, such as someone avoiding you because they assume you could be unstable, violent, or dangerous due to your mental illness. Self-judgment is also a possibility. A person who experiences stigma may be treated differently and excluded from many aspects of life that the rest of society takes for granted, resulting in marginalisation.

Prejudice and discrimination

Prejudice and discrimination regarding mental health injuries refer to the act of treating someone unfairly or differently because they have a mental health condition. Officers may become labelled by their illness, which leaves them vulnerable to prejudice and discrimination.

Coping with the effects of prejudice and discrimination is distressing and can exacerbate mental illness. Many people assert that dealing with this is even more challenging than managing the mental illness itself[13].

Is it any wonder, then, why most people grapple with broaching the subject of mental health, be it at home, socially, or particularly

12 http://scholar.lib.vt.edu/theses/available/etd-05162005-181537/
13 https://issuu.com/ifmsa-egypt/docs/mental_health_manual_2021_2022

in the workplace? Perhaps it's because we are hesitant to delve into the incredibly delicate fabric of humanity — the most sacred, highly personal aspect of our mental health. It requires significant emotional capacity to do so. Mental health is often elusive, subjective, and can be tricky to discuss. Dealing with the intimacy of mental health can be uncomfortable, complex, and confronting for many. Consequently, there is a reluctance among many to engage in such discussions.

The combination of exposure to traumatic experiences, an ingrained culture of distrust and cynicism, traditional masculine values, a warrior identity embodying resilience, personal sacrifice, courage, and strength, coupled with organisational injustices, all contribute to the elevated risk of law enforcement officers developing a mental illness.

It requires a specific type of individual to be exposed, day in and day out, to the continual and cumulative stresses of the job. To the community, law enforcement stereotypically symbolises authority, strength, integrity, and self-reliance; controlled emotions, and the capacity to handle complex problems. Officers are considered by the public to be imperturbable and unshakeable, seen as guardians and heroes.

> *'... I cannot talk about my mental health issues from work... I have struggled for many years... I am also gay and my country outlaws homosexuality... I can't afford to be exposed in any way...'*

Workplace social determinants

Beyond exposure to trauma, workplace and institutional social determinants, such as gender, age, ethnicity, socioeconomic status, race, status, culture, leadership, and sexual orientation, can significantly impact law enforcement officers' mental health. Other social conditions — such as interpersonal, family, and community dynamics, social support, employment opportunities, and work conditions — can further fuel and increase the propensity for heightened mental health risks.

Fear and shame

One of the most common reasons for not seeking help is fear and shame. Law enforcement officers view the world through a somewhat narrow social lens. Their exposure to poor mental health is often through dealing with individuals suffering severe psychological responses or significant behavioural disturbances. Consequently, law enforcement officers may associate the negativity of stigma and discrimination related to mental illness with their own potential mental health afflictions. Hence, their default position is often *'I don't want to be labelled as mentally ill or crazy'*. They immediately perceive such labelling as career-ending.

Lack of insight

As the saying goes, *'You don't know what you don't know'*. If you lack insight, understanding, or knowledge, how can you recognise the signs, indications, and behaviours of developing or possessing a mental health injury? How then can you help yourself or others?

Limited awareness

An individual may acknowledge some mental health concerns but lack full awareness of their significance. Alternatively, they may not understand that they have an actual illness. They might dismiss or minimise their issues, claiming, *'Everyone gets stressed out,'* *'My problems aren't that bad,'* or *'You're making more out of this than necessary.'*

Feelings of inadequacy

Many in law enforcement believe they are inadequate or a failure if they admit something is *'wrong'* with their mental health. Further, they often think they *'should be able to handle things'* on their own without help and that asking for assistance implies they are *'weak or inferior'*.

Distrust

Revealing personal details to a supervisor, doctor, psychologist, or counsellor can be challenging. Law enforcement officers often express concerns about *'telling a stranger'* about their problems. They worry that their personal information won't be kept confidential, and their department will be informed of their issues. Concerns regarding confidentiality in law enforcement are significant impediments to help-seeking behaviour. The notion that those who seek mental health services in law enforcement are unfit to serve remains a strong belief within the profession.

Hopelessness

Some individuals become demoralised by their mental health issues and believe *'nothing will help me'* or *'I'll never get better'*. Hopelessness is a significant mindset when injured. It permeates all facets of thinking, and in the early stages, you often can't see beyond what is happening to you. It often feels like you are the only one with this burden hanging over you.

Unavailability

Even if someone is interested in seeking mental health treatment, they may not know how to find appropriate professional care or are confused by the myriad information available on the internet. In some geographic areas, there may be few or limited mental health resources available.

Practical barriers

There is a growing body of evidence highlighting the importance of addressing barriers to help-seeking. Help-seeking is a critical part of mental health promotion and prevention, and early intervention is key to reducing the negative consequences of mental illness.

Several methods can overcome barriers to help-seeking. At the individual level, increasing education and knowledge about mental health and services, and improving communication skills can help overcome personal barriers. At the family level, increasing family support and communication and improving access to services and resources can help overcome family barriers. At the organisational level, increasing support and communication, and improving access to services and resources can help overcome barriers.

Another common barrier to mental health care is the inability to pay for treatment due to financial hardship or lack of health insurance. The lack of reliable transportation, childcare issues, and treatment appointments that conflict with work or school schedules can also prevent someone from engaging in treatment. The belief that mental health professionals cannot relate to those working in law enforcement jobs is also a substantial impairment for those seeking help.

It's important to note that overcoming barriers to help-seeking is a process, and there isn't a one-size-fits-all solution. What works for one person may not work for another, and what works for one family may not work for another. It's also vital to remember that overcoming barriers to help-seeking is an ongoing process, and there may be setbacks along the way.

✧

Chapter 8
Time Is Ticking

*'Every minute delayed, every hour wasted...every day
lostmeans another day we as leaders have failed those
we ask to answer the call of duty.'*
— Todd Doherty, MP Member of Parliament in the
House of Commons of Canada Cariboo—Prince George

Time is ticking; it is of the essence.

In recent years, the mental health of law enforcement officers has become an increasingly pressing issue. despite this escalating problem, law enforcement agencies have largely been passive in their response. Mental illness is often viewed as a taboo topic within the police force, with officers hesitant to seek help for fear of appearing weak or unfit for duty.

Some of the benefits of dealing with mental illness immediately include preventing the condition from getting worse and causing more harm to oneself or others, improving the quality of life and well-being of the injured and their loved ones, and increase the chances of recovery and reduce the risk of relapse.

Law enforcement agencies can no longer afford to be bystanders in the decline of their officers' mental health. They must take proactive measures to address the issue and support the individuals who prioritise service over self.

One approach involves improving access to mental health services. This includes having mental health professionals within the department and external referral sources. Officers should be able to seek help without fearing repercussions, and they need to know resources are available to them.

Another strategy is to expand training and education on mental health. This could help destigmatise mental health within the department, encouraging officers to seek help when needed, and equipping them to better understand and cope with their mental health challenges.

Lastly, law enforcement agencies need to foster a supportive and understanding culture towards mental health. This entails creating an environment where officers can discuss their mental health without fear of judgement or reprisal, supporting them when they take time off for mental health reasons, and accommodating their needs.

Diagnosing and treating physical health problems follow a well-accepted convention: identify the problem, seek a diagnosis, and begin treatment. For instance, if someone experiences persistent back pain, they would likely visit their general practitioner for treatment guidance[14]. However, the steps for mental health diagnosis and treatment are less clear-cut. Ambiguity exists from identifying signs of mental illness and the need for treatment, to knowing how or where to access treatment, to understanding that treatments are effective. Many individuals not only fail to recognise their mental health status but are often reluctant to seek a diagnosis due to stigma around mental illness and fear of discrimination. Often, it's a spouse or close family member who identifies the need for treatment and pressures their loved one to seek help.

---

14 https://www.ncbi.nlm.nih.gov/pmc/articles/PMC8408306/

Despite substantial efforts and increased investment in mental health service delivery in law enforcement, a significant unmet need for mental health services remains. If left untreated, mental health problems can worsen, resulting in severe negative impacts on all aspects of a person's life.

Indeed, what other profession demands dealing with humanity's worst? What other job requires a constant state of hypervigilance, yet the calmness to act as a counsellor, social worker, psychologist, medic, lawyer, teacher, or prison warden? What other profession allows you to take a person's liberty, or worse, use deadly force, but then mandates that you assist the person who just tried to harm or kill you? What job makes you question whether you'll return to your loved ones at the end of each day?

Mental health is not separate from the other dimensions of an individual's overall personal wellbeing; it is not insulated from the surrounding political, economic, material, and social conditions.

Until recently, the focus has primarily been on law enforcement suicide and peer support systems encouraging those suffering to seek help. Other social conditions, including interpersonal, family, and community dynamics, social support, employment opportunities, and work conditions, can also influence mental health risks and outcomes, both positively and negatively.

The inherent danger and unpredictability of law enforcement work is highly stressful, irrespective of one's rank or position, and places staff at risk of developing substantial physical illnesses. Conditions such as high blood pressure, insomnia, elevated levels of destructive stress hormones, and heart problems are just a few examples of the health issues faced.

A newly minted officer, having just graduated from the academy, is often in the best physical shape of their life. That young

'...One of my staff was struggling... I could see it and spoke with her... I wasn't sure what to do... but I knew that by just talking to her it might help. I came into work early one morning and saw that she had taken her own life... I was so distraught... my boss when he found out berated me, telling me that I knew she had been "sick" and said I should have done something... the worst was he looked me in the eye and told me it was all my fault she "had killed herself"...'

officer has also passed a psychological screening assessment, indicating good mental health. The tragedy is that over the next 20 to 25 years of their careers, these officers are likely to suffer physical illness and emotional trauma with devastating consequences[15]. When compared to their civilian counterparts, law enforcement officers not only have a shorter life expectancy but also higher rates of heart disease, hypertension, diabetes, and obesity. A career in law enforcement can also lead to higher instances of divorce, substance and alcohol abuse, and suicide. Their life expectancy is, on average, 22 years less than their civilian counterparts.

The mental illness of law enforcement officers must be prioritised, it can no longer be the 'elephant in the room' when discussing the profession's 'wellbeing'. It is a critical issue that can no longer be ignored. The time has come for law enforcement agencies to take proactive steps to support the men and women who put service before self.

Remember, if you, or someone you know are suffering, you are not alone and there is hope. Dealing with mental illness immediately can make a big difference in your life.

15 https://iamsigma.com/heart-disease-1-killer-of-active-and-retired-cops-1/

Chapter 9

How Can You Help Others If You Don't Look After Yourself First?

'Remember be good to yourself. If you don't,
take care of your body where are you going to live?'
— Kobi Yameda

I t is often said that you cannot help others if you do not help yourself first. This is especially true in leadership roles where you are responsible for others. If you are not looking after yourself, it will be difficult to lead others effectively.

There are a number of ways that you can help yourself as a leader. Firstly, it is important to set aside time for yourself. This can be used for anything from relaxation and rejuvenation to continuing education and personal development. It is important to have time where you are not focused on work or your responsibilities to others. This will help you maintain your energy and enthusiasm for your role.

Secondly, it is crucial to take care of your physical health. This means eating well, exercising regularly, and getting enough sleep.

When you are physically healthy, you will be better equipped to handle the demands of your role.

Thirdly, it is essential to look after your mental health. This entails taking time to relax and de-stress, as well as seeking help if you are feeling overwhelmed or struggling to cope. Mental health is just as important as physical health, and it is vital to care for both in order to be an effective leader.

Fourthly, having a support network is important. This can include family, friends, colleagues, or a professional network. These people can provide advice, guidance, and support when you need it. Having a support network will help you maintain balance in your role.

Finally, it is important to remember that you are not perfect. Leaders are often under a lot of pressure to be perfect, but this is not feasible. Everyone makes mistakes, and it is important to learn from them. Don't beat yourself up over minor errors; instead, learn from them to avoid making the same mistakes in the future.

Many years ago, as I began my journey towards being the best version of myself, I discovered the six pillars of health. These pillars form the foundation of my personal health strategy. Although their structure can vary, they are generally quite similar. However, it's important to recognise that they are individually developed and implemented. Just like any structure, without strong and stable pillars, most would collapse. These pillars guided me and allowed for meaningful progress in how I feel. They provided me with the tools to look within and establish what my body needs to respond to the stresses and chaos of everyday life. With these tools, I could aim at building self-mastery and self-trust to create a vibrant well-being that was tailor-made for me.

If you follow these tips, you will be better able to look after yourself and help others.

Nutrition and nourishment

Throughout my career, I was often encouraged to go with 'your gut feeling'. You know, that feeling of butterflies in your stomach or when the hairs on your neck rise up? These sensations emanating from your body suggest that your brain and gut are connected. It's a survival mechanism that can prepare you for the fight-or-flight response.

What's more, recent studies show that your brain affects your gut health and your gut may even affect your brain health. The communication system between your gut and brain is called the gut–brain axis, and if you fail to adequately fuel that nexus through good nutrition, you could potentially damage or limit the effectiveness of that relationship.

Nutrition embodies the concept of food as medicine and the idea that what we put into our system has the ability to heal or harm us. In our time, we often prefer the convenience of highly processed, simple fast foods to quickly quell our hunger pains, while continuing to meet our work obligations. Of course, there should be room in our life to experience these joys; however, like most things in life, moderation is best.

At the most basic level, nourishment is about eating real, whole foods – foods that don't need an ingredient list. Feed your body with a variety of amazing foods that come from the earth. You should aim to eat all the colours of the rainbow and consume food that isn't contaminated with pesticides, chemicals, or is highly processed.

'..I never really thought about how bad my eating habits were, I'd always eat quickly on the run and usually go for the most convenient, quick item, which was usually junk food.. no wonder I always felt terrible..'

It's crucial to eliminate foods that are toxic to your body — foods to which you're allergic or sensitive, foods full of chemicals difficult for your body to digest properly, and foods with unrecognisable ingredients.

Finally, nourishment includes how you eat: to maximise benefits, aim to eat mindfully, enabling your body to be in 'rest and digest' mode, absorbing all the amazing nutrients you're consuming. Take the time to truly savour your food by eating slowly, giving yourself a well-deserved break from life's turmoil.

Movement

Movement pertains to how you exercise and engage your body. We are designed to move and be active. However, our lives have become increasingly sedentary. Sitting is now referred to as the new 'smoking' by many medical practitioners due to its detrimental impact on our health. Importantly, this pillar is not about desperately burning calories by running 5–10 kilometres or sculpting the perfect physique through countless hours at the gym. Instead, it's about integrating movement into your daily life in a way that's sustainable, enjoyable, relaxing, and allows for a strong and capable body to carry you through your career and life.

I have reframed how I view exercise, shifting from it being a chore to a necessary practice. Exercise is no longer a 'nice to have' but a life necessity. Importantly, it's highly personalised. Take time to discover what kind of movement energises you and feels good in your body, rather than something that drains or uninspires you. Developing a consistent movement practice allows you to be genuine in your exercise endeavour, reclaiming it as part of your life, rather than an achievement or means to a false ideal. What matters is your consistent commitment to doing something.

Stress and fatigue management

An unfortunate part of the law enforcement job is that we are required to be 'on' all day, every day, and our nervous systems take a toll. I still struggle with hypervigilance, a state of increased alertness where I am extremely sensitive to my surroundings. It can make me feel like I'm constantly on alert for any hidden dangers, whether from other people or the environment. Often, though, these dangers are not real.

The elevated stress response impacts every area of health in the body. Internationally renowned researchers like Professor John Violanti, a law enforcement veteran who served as a New York state police trooper for 23 years, and Dr Kevin Gilmartin, a retired law enforcement officer from Arizona, USA, specialising in law enforcement and public safety-related issues, have extensively detailed this in their research.

Stress management comes in many forms — yoga, counselling, breathing, mindfulness, saying 'no', doing more things that bring joy, learning self-soothing skills, working less and playing more, eating nourishing food, talking to a friend, and so on. Winding down is about finding what works for you.

Sleep hygiene

Anyone who has worked in law enforcement knows that sleep often falls to the bottom of the priority list. I recall in my younger years as a police detective working beyond 24 hours straight, and occasionally going beyond 40 hours without sleep. Being so sleep-deprived is both physically and psychologically damaging.

Sleep is one of the building blocks of health; it is essential for all our biological processes, stable mental health, and is when a significant amount of repair in the body and brain occurs. If you aren't sleeping well, you will have a really hard time achieving your health goals. So, if you know that sleep isn't optimal, take the time to establish healthy habits around it; eat your last meal about three hours before going to bed, turn off screens at least two hours before going to sleep, go to sleep when you are tired, sleep in a dark and cool room, cut the alcohol, try taking a bath before bedtime or doing some gentle stretching or a restorative yoga class.

Connection

This pillar relates to your connection with yourself, others (community), and the natural world around you. I consider this to be one of the most important pillars. A sense of belonging is key to our spiritual self. I often refer to law enforcement as a global family, with which I am immediately comfortable despite jurisdictional, cultural, ethnic, or geographic differences. The trap for me was that over the decades, my social connectedness narrowed to only those in the job. It's crucial that we develop relationships with a few important people who truly know us, along with trust in our relationship with our internal emotional landscape.

However, before I could expand my social network, I had to develop a deep connection with myself to understand what feels good to me, my body, my values, and what my heart desired. I had to consider how I truly wanted to live my life and with whom I wanted to spend my time. Stress will persist indefinitely if you're living out of alignment. It's essential to understand what your most aligned self looks like, and follow that pathway to improved mental health, wellbeing, and harmony.

Connection, too, is a practice. My journey in this space continues, and I am learning how I can better myself using therapy, other spiritual (not religious) guidance, meditation, writing, mindfulness, and breathing, to name but a few. We experience connection when we hug another human, practice gratitude, commit random acts of kindness, and place our bare feet on the earth, wade through beach waters, or simply sit in the sun listening to the wind. Connection often requires intentionally slowing down, which can be challenging given the current pace of life. So, start small, assess your situation, establish a practice regime that suits your needs and desires, open your mind, and try different things to gauge what works and what doesn't for you.

Purpose/identity

Finding our purpose or identity is not a one-time event, but a lifelong journey. It may change over time as we grow, learn, and experience different things. It may also involve some uncertainty, risk, or failure along the way. However, by being open-minded, curious, and proactive, we can find more clarity, fulfillment, and joy in our lives.

There is no simple or definitive answer to this question, but there are some steps that can help us explore and discover our own unique purpose and identity.

One way is to reflect and ask yourself a series of questions like?

- What are my strengths and weaknesses?
- What are my passions and interests?
- What are my values and beliefs?
- What are my goals and aspirations?
- How do I cope with stress and challenges?
- How do I express myself creatively or artistically?
- How do I communicate and interact with others?
- How do I deal with conflict and disagreement?
- How do I handle feedback and criticism?
- How do I celebrate my achievements and successes?

From answering these questions, you can experiment and take action. You can try out different things that are of interest, challenge you, or make you curious. You can join clubs, take courses, start projects, or apply for jobs that relate more to your values, passions, or goals. You can also set specific and realistic objectives to work towards and measure your progress. By doing these things, you can learn more about yourself, your preferences, your abilities, and your potential. You can also discover new possibilities and directions that you may not have considered before.

Chapter 10
Wellness and Its importance

*'The concept of total wellness recognises that our every thought,
word, and behaviour affect our greater health and wellbeing.
And we, in turn, are affected not only emotionally but
also physically and spiritually.'*

— Greg Anderson

Health and wellness programs in law enforcement have traditionally focused on factors contributing to the alarming health consequences of the profession.

However, the terms 'health' and 'wellness' have often been used interchangeably and harmoniously for the sake of convenience. While the concept of health is widely understood, wellness isn't as clear. Regrettably, there's no universally accepted definition of wellness. Wellness is something you choose to pursue, not something that can be bestowed upon you. It's a life choice that requires constant effort and diligence to achieve, and it can be challenging to attain in a law enforcement career.

Although wellness is associated with a healthy lifestyle, it extends beyond the confines of general health. It encompasses a positive outlook on mind, body, and soul, and is typically within our control more than health. Wellness has various dimensions and can be viewed as a quality, state, or process.

Almost all wellness activities are proactive, not reactive. Instead of fixing a problem when it arises, wellness encourages continuous self-improvement. It's not about achieving your own ideas of perfection or meeting an unattainable benchmark. Instead, it's about caring for your complete self and consistently expanding your potential.

To simplify, wellness can be represented through a wellness wheel. This provides a visual representation of seven dimensions of wellness, allowing you to evaluate your performance in each category. Each wheel is individually created. For example, I've included my personal wellness wheel.

I regularly use the wellness wheel to reflect on my progress and understand what lifestyle adjustments I might need to make on my journey towards better health. Remember, though, the wellness wheel is an individual process, and what works for one person may not apply to another.

Here's how my six pillars form my wellness wheel:

1. Physical wellness

The physical dimension of the wellness wheel pertains to your body's health. It involves all types of physical activities, nutrition and balanced diets, sleep, strength, and seeking medical care when necessary.

Set some goals; they provide direction in achieving your aim and can boost motivation.

For many, exercising with a friend or colleague encourages physical activity and provides the added benefit of socialising. For others, like me, it means seeking solitude and quiet to focus and commit to your best efforts.

However, start small. Don't embark on a program suited for an elite or Olympic athlete. Keep perspective and remind yourself that merely starting a physical activity is an achievement.

Consistency in your effort is more sustainable and impactful for long-term commitment.

Vary your activities to keep things interesting; your body quickly adapts to activity, so regular change while keeping things fun and light can help you achieve this.

2. Emotional wellness

Also known as emotional health or wellbeing, emotional wellness refers to a person's ability to manage their emotions and the varied experiences they encounter throughout life. Are you in tune with your feelings so you can understand and express them? A solid foundation in emotional health equips you to adapt to life's changes and manage stress better.

Nurture your emotional wellness by getting enough sleep, checking in with a therapist when you can, much like a regular physical exam with your GP. Don't hesitate to ask for help when needed and regularly check in with yourself to manage overall stress.

Being unable to maintain a positive emotional state can lead to worsening outcomes, primarily because a negative emotional state is stressful.

Having strong emotional wellness can help you thrive. I've found numerous benefits of good emotional wellbeing: optimal relationships with others, reduced stress leading to less illness and increased immunity, positivity promoting productivity, and acknowledging your feelings to understand how you're truly feeling.

Initiate a self-care routine using whatever works for you. For me, meditation, grounding activities, stretching, or breathing exercises help calm my body and mind.

Be realistic when you're not feeling 100%. Certain times of the year may be more stressful than others, like holidays or certain anniversaries. It's important to prioritise your mental health, especially when you're not feeling your best, even if that means saying no to some things. You deserve to take care of yourself.

Learn to say no. Saying yes when you want to say no can leave you feeling resentful and overwhelmed. Establishing clear boundaries shows self-respect and care, and can help prevent resentments from building up.

3. Intellectual wellness

Intellectual wellness embodies a commitment to lifelong learning, fostering a desire to think critically and expansively. Cultivating your intellect is an invaluable tool, enabling the expansion of existing skills and knowledge, the development of new expertise, and enhancement of creativity, critical thinking, and problem-solving abilities. It encourages an enduring curiosity, learning, and participation in creative activities to keep your mind healthy and active.

Critical thinking abilities can enhance your leadership skills, especially in aspects such as time management and self-organisation. Clear thinking can aid in efficiently completing projects and combatting procrastination when you're able to clearly see the benefits of not leaving your work until the last minute.

Reading is a straightforward way to improve intellectual wellness. Dedicate time each day, even if it's just five minutes, to read for pleasure. You might read a few pages of an inspirational book in the morning while enjoying your coffee. Pleasure reading, keeping updated on social and political issues, or mentoring individuals all contribute to intellectual wellness.

Stimulating mental activities, from brain teaser apps to board games can help you keep your brain functioning well. When you play with other people, you're also bringing in a social aspect and, since humans are social animals, playing with others also increases intellectual wellness.

> *'...I opened the container doors and immediately recognised the smell...the smell of death. Sixteen people lay dead, including some young children... the scene was horrific...the smugglers had placed scented candles inside to disguise the faeces and urine smell...the sights and smells I was exposed to that day have never left me... I just carried on with my work like nothing out of the ordinary happened... but it did and I have since paid a heavy price.'*

Learning a new language is a highly brain-stimulating activity. When you learn a new language, you induce changes in your brain's anatomy, which includes reshaping your functional neural patterns and enhancing neuroplasticity.

I found reading to be invaluable in expanding my knowledge and understanding of mental health, particularly how it impacted me, my colleagues, family, and friends.

Compile a list of topics that intrigue you. To foster your intellectual wellness, maintain a record of captivating topics and devote some time each month to further research.

Setting aside daily time to jot down your thoughts and ideas is a remarkable way to stimulate your intellect.

4. Spiritual wellness

Before you can improve your spiritual wellness, it's crucial to comprehend what it is. Spiritual wellness is the process by which you search for meaning and purpose in life. It can be achieved through various means, including organised religion, prayer, meditation, yoga, as well as a thoughtful evaluation of your morals, values, ethics, and beliefs.

Spiritual wellness is important for several reasons. Firstly, it enables you to contemplate your life's purpose and solidify your 'why'. We are all here for a reason. Some of us identify that reason earlier than others. However, taking the time to explore your purpose and understand why you do the things you do is a robust foundation for leading a meaningful life.

Spiritual wellness is crucial as it enables us to clear our minds and accept the things that are beyond our control. The truth is, we exist in a fast-paced, chaotic world that's becoming more complex each day. Having the capacity to detach from the world and accept that what happens is often beyond your control is an empowering life skill.

5. Environmental wellness

Environmental wellness pertains to your feeling of safety, comfort, and connection with your physical surroundings. It encompasses the interactions between your environment, your community, and yourself. From a micro level within your own home to a global scale, our physical environment impacts our mental health, significantly affecting our mood and lifestyle. Environmental wellness focuses on how you interact with your surroundings, such as your home, school, or workspace.

Consider creating a healthy, inviting living space and assessing your personal living and workspace. What is pleasing to your eyes and what irritates you? Compile a list of manageable, tangible steps you could take to improve your space. You might declutter, add more colour, or introduce more light.

You could seek out small pockets of tranquillity by taking a moment out of your busy day to appreciate your surroundings. You can do this anywhere, but it's especially enjoyable in your favourite peaceful place.

6. Social wellness

Social wellness is defined as our ability to care for others while also taking good care of ourselves, a critical aspect of successful leadership.

The relationships we establish can greatly affect the quality of our lives. Our ability to form meaningful connections with others – as a family, a society, and a community – is referred to as social wellness.

The social wellness dimension of the wellness wheel relates to the quality of your relationships with others. Maintaining a strong network of individuals to whom you feel connected is key to your social wellness, and can help ward off feelings of stress, isolation, loneliness, or even depression.

7. Occupational wellness

According to the World Health Organisation (WHO), most individuals spend one-third of their adult life at work. Assuming another third is spent sleeping (given they're receiving enough rest), this represents a significant amount of time! Therefore, comprehending what occupational wellness is, its importance, and how to enhance it, is crucial to your workplace satisfaction[16].

Before you can improve your occupational wellness, it's essential to understand what it entails. In essence, occupational wellness relates to maximising your workplace satisfaction by focusing on work that elicits feelings of joy, fulfilment, and accomplishment. It can be achieved by exploring various career pathways and effectively managing workplace stressors.

Separate work from home. As challenging as it can sometimes be, endeavour to avoid excessive overlap between work

---

16 https://www.who.int/news-room/fact-sheets/detail/spending-on-health-a-global-overview

responsibilities and your home life. If you work from home, attempt to establish a distinct space for work hours, like a desk or workstation that you can leave when you wish to relax or spend time with loved ones.

Socialise at work. Feeling connected to your co-workers is important. A great way to socialise and get to know each other better is by catching up during breaks, learning about their hobbies, likes, and dislikes.

Ask for feedback. As leaders, we excel at providing feedback to staff. Aim to deliver feedback positively; avoid negativity or demeaning comments, which I find can be counterproductive. Regularly seek feedback, not only during performance evaluations. I found it immensely rewarding to seek feedback from the staff I oversaw. Though many considered my request unconventional and were concerned about offending 'the boss', true leadership involves accepting both positive and negative feedback. While the feedback was confronting at times, upon reflection and self-analysis, I found meaning that allowed me to grow and adapt my style.

Take mental health days. Remember to check in with yourself to avoid burnout and communicate openly with your boss about your mental health. An occasional day off can boost productivity and provide time and space to focus on mental health. As a leader, this sets a wonderful example to your staff that you practice what you preach. This has a significant impact and empowers them to ask for the same, confident they won't be condemned or ridiculed.

Communicate. Discuss with your co-workers and supervisors how you're truly performing at work and don't hesitate to ask for additional support when needed. I've found that showing vulnerability is a powerful tool, demonstrating to your staff that you're human too, and not immune from life's and work's stressors. It is a true sign of compassion and sets a wonderful standard that influences others to do likewise.

How can you improve occupational wellness?

Firstly, setting professional goals is one of the most effective ways to enhance your occupational wellness. Whether broad or specific, writing down career goals, both immediate and aspirational, greatly increases your likelihood of working purposefully and following through with them.

Another way to improve occupational wellness is by seeking out mentors. Having someone who can offer professional guidance and career advice is invaluable. Mentors don't have to be directly involved in your organisation; in fact, it can often be beneficial to find mentors outside your organisation. Plus, they're likely to have experience with many of the challenges and obstacles you'll encounter throughout your career.

Lastly, commit to maintaining a strong work-life balance and always living in the present. In other words, learn to switch off from work! This includes making time for hobbies, social activities, and holidays.

By committing to developing your personal wellness wheel, you will have reflected deeply and introspectively, formulating strategies and ideas on how to improve your life, that of your family, and those whom you lead. It's a win-win situation.

✧

Chapter 11

IN TRUE LEADERSHIP, PEOPLE MATTER

'Nobody cares how much you know,
until they know how much you care.'
— Theodore Roosevelt, former US president
and New York City Police Commissioner

As previously noted, many in the law enforcement community are quite wary when it comes to seeking any form of mental health help. They often fear that doing so will make them appear weak, untrustworthy, unfit to continue in their role, and most significantly, put their job at risk. Numerous organisations worldwide are yet to acknowledge, let alone offer support for, their employees' mental health. When recognition does exist, the justification for this fear is often deeply rooted in official governance and policy.

Some agencies require officers seeking or receiving mental health treatment, or those taking, medications for treatment, to disclose this fact. They may then potentially face operational restrictions while under professional care. This type of stigma or misunderstanding perpetuates false information and traps law enforcement officers in a cycle of depression or anxiety. Rather than coming forward to seek help, many choose to suffer alone and in silence. However, they should never have to feel or act this way.

As a leader, it's highly likely that at some point in your career, you'll supervise a worker with mental illness, whether you're aware of it or not. A worker may develop mental illness before or during employment. Most workers successfully manage their illness without it affecting their work. Some may require workplace support for a short period, while others will need ongoing workplace strategies.

It's often presumed that a worker's mental illness develops outside of the workplace. However, an 'unhealthy' work environment or a workplace incident can cause considerable stress and exacerbate, or contribute to, the development of mental illness.

Addressing mental health in the workplace can be incredibly challenging, whether you're experiencing it yourself or are responsible for another employee. Unfortunately, mental health remains one of the toughest issues to discuss in a work environment. Balancing your professional obligations with your personal wellbeing can be stressful, and there is still a stigma associated with suffering from a mental health problem.

A question often asked by many law enforcement professionals is, *'What can I do to support and encourage staff to come forward if they're suffering?'*

The first step in normalising mental health in the workplace is knowing the signs that an employee may be struggling with. These signs can include withdrawing from their work or social circles, appearing not to be themselves, performance issues such as missing deadlines or a decline in work quality, absenteeism or unexplained absences from work, or showing up to work when an employee can't perform at their best, or acting erratically or being irritable.

So how do you start the conversation?

How are you?

We hear this question a dozen times every day. However, it's likely that our response seldom strays from the usual, 'Fine thanks, how about you?'

It can seem like we're caught in a never-ending conversational loop, repeating the same programmed response rather than expressing how we genuinely feel.

So, how do you answer when you're not okay? How do you tell a colleague that you've been in a dark place for a while now or that your anxiety is spiralling out of control? Like many, you probably don't want to burden others with your deeply personal problems.

How to ask?

So, let's say that you sense something's off with a colleague. Before you approach them, look for any signs of distress or unusual behaviour. Perhaps they've become more withdrawn and are drinking more than they typically do, or something just seems amiss. How do you check in on them? How do you move past these automatic responses and discover what's genuinely happening? Sometimes it's easy to discern that a colleague is having a rough time. Maybe they've recently experienced a devastating break-up, a chronic illness is flaring up, or they're facing issues at work. With this sort of stress on their plate, you may already suspect (or know) that they're not in a good place.

But other times, it's not so obvious.

However, there are other tell-tale signs to look out for. Keep an eye out for noticeable changes in their demeanour or appearance. For instance, maybe they've become withdrawn and aren't keeping in touch with coworkers or friends. Or perhaps they're looking more dishevelled and tired than usual. If something seems out of the ordinary, it likely is, so check in.

Ensure the time is right

There's a time and place for this kind of conversation. Ideally, you might put away your devices, brew a cuppa, and create a cosy spot where your workmate should feel comfortable enough to open up. Even if you're checking in virtually, choose a time when they can chat without distractions like work, childcare, or other commitments. If you're meeting in person, select a spot that's away from large crowds, loud noises, and is relatively private. Sometimes, taking a slow walk outside away from distractions is worth considering.

Make sure you're ready

Sharing your deepest personal thoughts takes a lot, and it can feel particularly exposing if they're dark or distressing. It's essential that you're in the right headspace to initiate this conversation. After all, when you're asking someone to be vulnerable, you want to ensure you're present in the conversation, attentive, and focused on what you're about to embark on.

Focus on the neutral

Knowing that you could quickly affect someone's mood with one simple, empathetic question shouldn't deter you from speaking to your workmate. The key to success is knowing how to communicate to show you care. Even if they're struggling, you don't want to exacerbate their situation.

The best way to find out if someone is okay is to allow them to talk about themselves. Ask friendly, open-ended questions without being condescending. If your workmate wants to talk, they will do so when you provide them with a neutral opening.

Neutral questions to ask

Instead of asking if your colleague is okay, asking neutral questions will offer opportunities for honest conversation. When you ask someone if they are okay, they can respond with a flat 'no', thus ending the discussion. If you want to talk and listen, provide neutral and open-ended prompts.

Starting with 'How's it going?' allows your colleague to answer honestly. This type of question is open to any response. No matter the answer you get, you can also follow it up with the statement, 'Tell me more'. Hopefully, your colleague will, and you can get to what is bothering them.

There's nothing condescending about 'How's it going?' because people use this question in many social settings. It's appropriate to ask anyone at almost any time. It's not offensive in the least. And it can be answered with single words or lengthy descriptions.

The other question that offers endless answers is, 'What are you up to these days?' If your colleague says 'nothing', then you'll want to ask, why? If your colleague provides an answer that is more than that, ask them to tell you more. Hopefully, your colleague will notice how interested you are and will open up to tell you what's happening in their lives.

Speak with care

This is a delicate conversation, so it's best to tread carefully. Consider what you're going to say beforehand. No one enjoys being interrogated. Remember, as law enforcement, you're trained to interview and extract information from people, but these techniques may not necessarily apply when speaking with someone suffering from mental health issues. You don't want to inadvertently blurt out something condescending or harmful. Instead, try saying something like, 'You know I care about you and I'm worried. I've noticed you've not been yourself lately'.

Ask twice

Admitting you're not okay is tough. Extremely tough. Therefore, it's understandable that someone might find it hard to open up straight away. If you suspect someone is struggling, asking twice could make a significant difference. Gently prod them by asking something as simple as 'Are you sure you're okay?', and follow it up with an example, something you've noticed in their behaviour. This signals to them that you know them well, and it shows that you're genuinely there for them and ready to lend a listening ear.

Listen carefully and without judgment

We've all been there. We've bared our soul to someone, shared our worries and fears, and they've awkwardly scrambled to find the right words to solve our problems. But sometimes things aren't fixable. Sometimes there's no magic solution or quick fix that can make everything better, and nothing you say could erase the pain they're feeling. You don't have to have all the answers. So don't ramble. Ensure you're genuinely listening to what they're saying. Because just being there for them could be all the help they need.

Active listening is crucial. It involves focusing entirely on the speaker, understanding their message, comprehending the information, and responding thoughtfully. Unlike passive listening, which entails hearing a speaker without retaining their message, this highly valued interpersonal communication skill ensures you're able to engage and later recall specific details without needing to repeat information. Active listening helps others feel comfortable sharing information with you. When you demonstrate your ability to sincerely listen to what others have to say, it builds trust. When people know they can speak freely to you without interruptions or judgement, they're more likely to confide in you.

Treat people with compassion

Compassion is the most essential skill needed when supporting someone who might be suffering from a mental health problem. Compassion involves recognising suffering in others and taking steps to help alleviate their discomfort. This may seem an odd requirement for law enforcement, as empathy and warmth run counter to the notion that in this profession, we must toughen up, set feelings aside, and maintain a steely demeanour to stay safe and catch criminals.

Maintaining compassion and empathy in a law enforcement career can prove challenging. Many officers face numerous crises and unique situations that can negatively affect their ability to cope with and uphold their sense of compassion. This harmful effect can lead officers to develop a void of compassion.

Trust your instinct and act on it. However, doing so requires understanding and skills.

> *'My job was as a forensic officer. Almost every day of my career, I would deal with death. I was okay with that. What I wasn't okay with was how my organisation banished me when I became sick with PTSD. Instead of helping me, they pensioned me out. I still haven't forgive them.'*

Compassion and empathy are inherently important to us as humans and to officers in particular. There are several distinct steps you can take to show compassion to others. They might include:

Firstly, practice self-compassion

Most of us, particularly in law enforcement, are our own harshest critics. Self-criticism can be a useful tool for self-growth;

however, when overused, it can also be highly destructive. If your inner voice is berating you for your inevitable imperfections, you'll find it challenging to show compassion to others when they reveal their humanity. Accept that both you and others are human and imperfect.

Move beyond self-referencing

From the time we're children, many of us are taught, 'It's all about me'. But in reality, we're all connected. Practise shifting your perspective away from solely thinking about how something affects you. This doesn't mean neglecting yourself to please someone else — that's not self-compassion! Instead, it means expanding your awareness to make room for the interconnectedness that unites us all.

Be empathetic

There's a difference between being sympathetic and empathetic. Being empathetic means that we put ourselves in the other person's shoes. It doesn't mean you have to have been in jail or been poor to understand the plight of those experiencing it. But you can try to understand the other person's feelings.

Empathy starts with listening and ends with seeing the world through the other person's eyes. Sympathy is just feeling sorry for someone without the effort to understand. We can show the most compassion by being empathetic.

Respect boundaries

Make it your duty to respect people's wishes. By doing this, you're conveying that you respect their boundaries. If your co-worker declines your help, respectfully accept it and don't push further. Importantly, don't take it personally. That's perhaps the most compassionate thing you can do under the circumstances.

You've done nothing wrong. Pride and not feeling deserving of kindness can cause some individuals to refuse help.

Offer hope

Telling someone, 'It's going to get better', is one way to inspire hope. However, making promises that potentially can't be kept could be devastating for someone with a mental health issue. A better option might be to assure them that you're there for them, which is a more appropriate thing to say. If you over-promise and under-deliver, trust will be eroded.

Being able to express compassion in the workplace requires the ability to know your colleagues and staff. It is valuable to get to know those you work with and who work for you, such as their birthdays, outside interests, and the names of their spouses, children, or loved ones. While these can be helpful starting points, truly attempting to understand your colleagues, rather than superficially getting to know them, will have a deeper, far-reaching impact.

> I recall a time when I was in Timor-Leste, helping to strengthen the young nation's police establishment. I would informally meet with each of the staff who worked for me, including the locally engaged staff; that is, those Timorese who worked alongside me. Most were terrified that 'the boss' wanted to see them and thought they were in some sort of trouble. But after explaining that was not the case, and that all I wanted to do was get to know them, we would just chat. This simple act had a substantial impact on the individuals by making them feel valued, but it also allowed me time to understand them. Things such as, are they more of a loner or social? Do they prefer email, instant messaging, or face-to-face communication? Or a combination of all of them?

Understanding their work routine and their preferences is important. Do they cope well with uncertainty, or are they risk-averse, preferring planning and a more predictable work environment?

Are they talkative and social or are they a more introverted or private type? Are they career-driven, or do they enjoy their hobbies outside of work more?

You might think that this is all 'soft' leadership stuff. But in my experience, taking an interest in the people you lead will help you build trust, especially if the time came to engage them if they weren't feeling right.

✧

Chapter 12

Leadership — Influence What You Can When You Can

'To improve is to change; to be perfect is to change often.'
— Winston Churchill

Leadership styles are as diverse as the individuals that embody them. Some leaders are born; others are nurtured. Some are charismatic, while others are not. Some leaders act ethically, while others fall short. In the realm of leadership, three terms — ethical, authentic, and moral — are frequently interchanged, despite their distinct differences.

Ethical leadership hinges on a moral code, emphasising the importance of acting rightly, even when it's challenging or against the crowd. Authentic leadership revolves around authenticity, underscored by genuineness, honesty, and transparency. Meanwhile, moral leadership emphasises integrity, doing what is right, even when unobserved.

Each leadership style holds significant weight. Ethical leadership shapes the organisation's overall tone, as unethical leadership can cultivate a similar environment. Authentic leadership fosters trust, crucial for any follower-leader relationship. Moral leadership sets the standard for others to emulate.

Leaders who embody ethical, authentic, and moral leadership are often the most effective. These leaders earn trust through consistently acting right, being genuine and honest, and leading with integrity.

Regrettably, many recent leaders have shown significant ethical or moral deficiencies, impacting their employees' overall wellbeing. As a leader, I've observed these shortcomings first-hand and initiated changes to counteract them, using a vision-guided approach, and fostering engagement and commitment from my team.

My leadership style leans heavily towards ethical, authentic, and moral dimensions. This style, known as values-based leadership, stays true to my core principles. Although open to altering strategies, plans, and work style, I consistently uphold my principles, values, and ethics.

Positive values-based leadership emphasises ethical and moral decision-making. This approach cultivates a positive work environment, inspiring employees to excel. By stressing the significance of positive values, leaders can foster trust and respect within their organisations. This approach encourages collaboration, as shared values promote cooperation. Additionally, it enhances employee loyalty and commitment, with shared beliefs fostering a deeper connection to the organisation. Lastly, it paves the way for a culture of success, with ethical behaviour promoting productivity.

Positive values-based leadership goes beyond leveraging strengths and creating meaning. It involves engaging employees, helping them flourish personally and professionally, boosting productivity, creativity, and financial returns. Success evaluated based on values is the best way to foster a high-performance culture[17].

17 https://www.researchgate.net/publication/331659641_Leadership_Values_and_
Values_Based_Leadership_What_is_the_Main_Focus

Values-based leadership rests on four principles: self-reflection, balance, true self-confidence, and genuine humility. These are key in regaining and maintaining trust[18].

Introducing a values-based leadership program can catalyse the development of an organisational culture centred on empathy. Greater understanding of our colleagues paves the way for more meaningful work relationships, reduced health issues like stress, burnout, and compassion fatigue, and a more contented, productive, and harmonious workplace.

However, employees may not be willing to discuss their mental health if your office hasn't actively fostered a culture of connection and psychological safety — where they can feel safe to openly express themselves and discuss the challenges they may be facing.

For a fulfilling work environment, individuals must feel a sense of belonging, importance, and appreciation from their organisation. Without these elements, workplaces can become breeding grounds for isolation and aggravate mental health issues. As a leader, displaying consistent empathy and understanding is crucial, fostering an environment where employees feel safe addressing workplace stressors.

However, even within an open work culture, there's often apprehension about discussing mental health issues, particularly when the work environment contributes to these challenges.

As a leader, it is vital to consider the impact your actions and decisions have on your team. This doesn't suggest shying away from difficult decisions, but instead ensuring minimal distress is imposed on your staff. Be cognisant that you might unintentionally be a stressor for your team, possibly by exerting undue

---

18 http://archive.sciendo.com/ARHSS/arhss.2018.15.issue-1/arhss-2018-0005/
   arhss-2018-0005.pdf

pressure, making unrealistic demands, or abruptly changing priorities. To prevent this, actively encourage feedback and be open to receiving it.

One of the most effective methods I've employed to solicit feedback is integrating it into performance-management discussions. Following the formal evaluation of staff, I would ask, 'How am I performing? Am I providing the support you need? Is there anything I can do to alleviate your stress?' The impact of this simple question on my team was remarkable. It often took them by surprise that I would even consider asking such a question. However, they unanimously agreed that this small gesture significantly improved their work experience and, most importantly, fostered an open and trusting relationship.

Leaders may understandably struggle to balance empathy for an employee facing mental health challenges with maintaining workplace accountability. If an employee is grappling with their mental health, it doesn't necessitate lowering your standards. However, some 'renegotiation' may be required to allow the employee to meet their responsibilities within their current health constraints. This balance is a challenge that many leaders grapple with.

> *'...When I was an inspector, I was leading a team at a major demonstration that became violent. We had urine and faeces thrown at us. We were spat at, had metal chairs and plastic barriers thrown at us. Some demonstrators were badly injured and we had to help them. One died. At the conclusion, I wanted to take my team to a quiet, secure space to talk about it. My boss told me, "No, that's not what we do. Back to work".'*

For example, an employee might need to adjust their work hours or spend more time working remotely to better handle mental health needs. Embrace this opportunity to show compassion, but also be clear and direct about expectations and responsibilities and do so empathetically.

By providing support to your employees, you empower them to maintain control as effectively as possible. This approach positively influences their recovery processes. As long as the standard of work is maintained, you should be open to making necessary adjustments, particularly given that flexible work arrangements have been shown to improve mental health. Demonstrate your care by regularly 'checking in' on their wellbeing before discussing their work progress. Additionally, use technology to provide opportunities for remote participation in team meetings and other activities when possible.

The following encapsulate the fundamental principles of ethical leadership[19]:

Respect: Respect in the workplace is essential. Leaders need to respect both themselves and their colleagues, acknowledging others' ideas, feelings, and principles. Differences of opinion are common in the workplace, but respect enables people to relate cordially despite these differences.

Justice: Ethical leaders must strive for fairness, treating everyone equally. For example, if a penalty for lateness exists, it should apply to all employees. This principle ensures no employees are treated unjustly.

Honesty: This is a critical ethical leadership principle. It entails being truthful, forthright, and transparent in all actions. An honest leader encourages employees to be equally open and truthful.

---

19 https://study.com/learn/lesson/ethical-leadership-principles-examples.html

Ethical leaders will not resort to dishonest actions, such as theft, to circumvent challenging situations.

Community: An ethical leader values the input of everyone involved, considering their suggestions and interests. Creating a sense of community within an organisation might include conducting surveys or team-building activities that allow employees to contribute to enhancing the workplace environment. Senior management should not make all decisions without involving other staff members.

Protection: Ethical leaders play a crucial role in ensuring the welfare of their employees. If working conditions in a department are subpar, an ethical leader will raise the issue with senior management rather than disregarding employees' complaints. It's critical that leaders meet the needs of their employees in order to achieve organisational goals.

Integrity: This is the capacity to stick to one's moral principles and values. Even when faced with tempting situations, a person with integrity remains honest and accountable, even when unobserved. Organisations prosper under leaders with integrity, as this helps to minimise financial losses.

Balancing mental health needs with workplace demands can be a complex task for leaders. To overcome mental health stigmas and foster an environment where every employee can thrive, leaders must recognise their role in addressing their team's mental health needs. By nurturing a compassionate, caring, and safe workplace culture that still emphasises accountability, you can create an environment where everyone can succeed while maintaining their mental health.

✦

Chapter 13

Leadership – It is Better to be Supportive than A Superior

'Become the kind of leader that people would follow voluntarily, even if you had no title or position.'

— Brian Tracy

Whether we realise it or not, we all embody some form of leadership in life. You might be leading a family, captaining a sports team, directing a workplace team, heading a department, or running a corporation — in all these situations, leadership is crucial. This is particularly true within law enforcement, where the public automatically perceives you, a law enforcement officer, as a leader, regardless of your rank, position, or skill level. You are leaders within your community.

In terms of leadership style, it is often more beneficial to be supportive rather than superior, as this encourages collaboration and cooperation among team members. A supportive leader is more likely to cultivate an environment of trust and under-standing, thereby fostering a positive atmosphere where team members feel comfortable taking risks and trying new things. By being supportive, a leader can also help their team develop their skills and abilities, leading to greater success in the long run.

Furthermore, adopting a supportive stance rather than a superior one allows a leader to build stronger relationships with their team members, which can help forge a stronger bond among them. Ultimately, being supportive rather than superior benefits both the leader and their team by encouraging collaboration, building trust, and promoting skill development.

Leadership has perhaps the most significant influence over the law enforcement workforce and its organisation. Any change in perceptions of mental healthcare, or attitudes towards people with mental illness among the workforce, can only occur when leadership champions the cause and filters this intention down through the organisation. It is the leaders who need to understand the necessity for this shift in mindset among their workforce, both from the organisation's benefit perspective and its social responsibility.

One of the lessons I've gleaned throughout my career is that leadership is a somewhat fluid principle. Most leaders adapt their styles to suit their situation. The longer they lead and the more they engage with their employees, the more they adapt and evolve their leadership style.

However, my experiences have also shown me that many individuals who successfully climb the promotional ladder are proficient parrots. By this, I mean they can accurately regurgitate, mimic, and espouse all aspects of what leadership entails. But, when you scratch the surface, you often find many of these individuals to be shallow and hollow, merely pretending to be leaders with little underlying substance.

Education in leadership has traditionally focused on five core leadership styles: benign, transformational, delegative, authoritative, transactional, and participative. These styles have largely remained unchallenged over decades, resulting in somewhat of a stall in the evolution of leadership capabilities.

'...It was Christmas eve...we were called to a head-on motor vehicle accident up on the highway... when we arrived, one car was on fire... we couldn't save the occupants... when the fire was extinguished... four bodies... two adults and two children were still in their seats...charred... their Christmas presents in the back were things that survived.... back then we had no debrief... no support...just had to "tough it out"...'

Leadership development tends to be inward-looking, dominated by normative models that prescribe what leaders ought to do. The focus is usually on individual attributes, traits, and competencies. However, in response to complexity, we need innovation, experimentation, and the leveraging of diverse thoughts, ideas, and experiences[20].

As a leader, it's critically important to understand your individual leadership style. You must grasp who you are, what's important to you, and comprehend the impact you have on yourself and those you influence directly.

Leaders need to be aware of their core values, understanding which aspects are fluid and which are non-negotiable. Without this foundational platform, how can a leader develop their unique style and technique?

If leaders have identified and shared their values with their teams, and demonstrate these values in their daily actions, they will establish trust visibly. Acting contrary to one's stated values can inflict lasting damage to trust, particularly in an organisation already suffering from high levels of distrust.

'Walk the talk' is perhaps the most significant advice for a leader. It is how you demonstrate your trustworthiness and showcase your ethical and principled leadership.

---

20 https://www.researchgate.net/publication/288887676_Police_Leadership_for_ Complex_Times

It's important to note that we can't find solutions to mental health issues by looking to the past, where solutions for physiological problems may have been successful. Mental health issues have unique nuances, as the social environment significantly impacts the decisions of people with these challenges. We need to find solutions that are far more inclusive and capable of fostering social transformation.

Leaders have a responsibility to communicate to their workforce that creating a supportive environment for those with mental health issues is everyone's task. Leadership needs to emphasise that when it comes to mental health, every employee is a stakeholder. It is only in the presence of an inclusive environment that staff with mental health challenges will feel encouraged to make the right decisions.

For many, the treatment they receive from their direct supervisor and the behaviour of the organisation's leaders significantly influences how they perceive themselves and their work. An abusive, negative, inconsistent, or disorganised manager can cause employees to suffer from stress-related health problems. Indeed, research shows that lack of managerial support is one of the most commonly cited factors in stress, anxiety, and depression. On the other end of the spectrum, feeling valued and supported by a manager can help individuals manage all kinds of difficulties, including mental health issues that could otherwise impede their performance.

Beyond their direct impact on employee mental health, managers and leaders can act as 'gatekeepers' to working conditions that either mitigate or amplify risks to employee mental well-being. This might involve preventing an unfair workload being placed on an individual or ensuring that organisational change is well communicated.

Line managers can also play a key role in early identification of mental health issues within their team. If an individual is experiencing a mental health issue, resolution is more likely if the manager is involved in finding a solution[21].

The first step to becoming an influential leader is understanding that leadership is more than just a position and making a conscious decision to be someone worth following. For law enforcement, this includes being a strong mental health leader.

Regrettably, little literature exists on how best to address mental health in the workplace specifically in relation to law enforcement education and development. While a plethora of books, articles, podcasts, and blogs discuss nearly every aspect of self-help and leadership, very few publications address the capacity of leaders to understand, support, and drive better mental health in the workplace.

Mental health awareness is a crucial leadership skill that is often overlooked but is vital for the long-term success of any organisation. As a leader, having a deep understanding of your team and a sensitivity to their well-being is essential. A team cannot work effectively if any of its members are grappling with personal challenges that bleed into their work-life without receiving support. Companies also have a responsibility to their staff to provide a positive working environment and to ensure that their work isn't causing mental or physical harm.

Leaders can profoundly impact the wellbeing of their staff. Being an effective leader for mental health involves developing exceptional emotional intelligence (EQ). EQ refers to the ability to identify and regulate our own emotions, recognise the emotions of others, empathise with them, and utilise these skills to communicate effectively and build healthy, productive

---

21 https://www.personneltoday.com/hr/managing-mental-health-work-role-leaders-line-managers/

83

relationships. Not only are these healthy, productive relationships key to psychological well-being, they also contribute to physical health.[22].

Fortunately, emotional intelligence isn't merely an inherent trait, something you either possess or lack. If you commit yourself to the task, you can learn the skills necessary to improve your emotional intelligence.

Leaders are best positioned to both identify mental health issues in workers and to respond to them in appropriate, meaningful ways. To earn the trust and confidence of their staff, it's crucial for leaders to have a basic understanding of mental health conditions, symptoms, and behaviours that could indicate potential issues, enabling early intervention strategies, just as they would for a physical injury[23].

Understanding the variety of trauma and operational stress issues that regularly confront law enforcement is essential in this context:

- **Acute trauma** – This is often associated with a single event in one's life.
- **Cumulative trauma** – This refers to adversity that arises from a lifetime exposure to an array of potentially traumatic events.
- **Compassion fatigue** – This is a condition characterised by a gradual lessening of compassion over time. It's common among workers who directly assist victims of trauma.
- **Vicarious trauma** – This results from empathetic engagement with traumatised individuals and their reports of traumatic experiences.

---

22 https://www.health.harvard.edu/mind-and-mood/emotional-intelligence
23 https://www.policechiefmagazine.org/the-divergence-of-institution-leadership-culture/

- **Operational stress injury** – This refers to any persistent psychological difficulty arising from operational duties.
- **Burnout** – This is defined as the harmful physical and emotional responses that occur when the job demands do not match the capabilities, resources, or needs of the worker.
- **Moral injury** – This emphasises the psychological, social, cultural, and spiritual aspects of trauma. Moral injury is a normal human response to an abnormal traumatic event. In the context of law enforcement, this could occur when officers witness or participate in events that violate their deeply held moral beliefs and expectations. Moral injury can also result from experiencing betrayal or transgressions within the workplace, leading to feelings of anger. It can affect those who have seen and experienced death, mayhem, destruction, and violence, thereby shattering their worldviews.

Show them you do truly understand.

Therefore, by embodying your principles, maintaining transparency, educating yourself on mental health, upholding values and ethics, and staying true to yourself, you demonstrate to those you lead that you understand and are compassionate about their well-being and mental health.

✧

Chapter 14

Leadership Can Be Draining

'A bad leader can take good staff and destroy them, causing the best employees to flee and the remainder to lose all motivation.'
— Unknown

Why can leadership be so draining?
There are a few different schools of thought when it comes to the idea of leadership being draining. The first belief is that leadership is a privilege and should not be taken for granted. This suggests that those in leadership positions should be aware of the significance their title carries and the responsibility they have towards those they are leading. The second belief posits that leadership is a demanding job and can often be taxing on those in the role. This is because leaders are often required to make difficult decisions, work long hours, and deal with significant stress. The third belief is that leadership is not inherently draining but can become so if the leader is not adequately supported. However, with proper support, leadership can be an immensely rewarding experience. This suggests that it's crucial for leaders to have a robust support system in place to avoid feeling overwhelmed by their responsibilities.

It's important that you take care of yourself whilst managing the pressures and responsibilities that come with such a role. By taking care of yourself, you can perform better as a leader, be more accessible, approachable, and effective. Thus, spending time on your mental health, though it may feel selfish, is not a self-indulgent exercise.

Here are some tips that will help you function at your best:

Be aware of your emotions and act accordingly – You hopefully wake up in a positive frame of mind, primed for a successful day, but we all know this isn't always the case. As hard as we try, personal and professional issues follow us throughout the day, affecting our emotions and functioning. If you've had a rough night with unwell kids or you're not feeling your best for whatever reason, consider whether the daily plan is still appropriate. The same goes for your team. Is today the best day to try changing a team member's behaviour when they are clearly struggling? It's not about making excuses or procrastinating; it's about understanding your team and considering outside pressures when managing them.

Know when you are at your best and schedule accordingly – Are you a morning person, or does it take a few hours for you to hit your stride? Are you more productive after hours when the rest of the team has left, the phones have stopped ringing, and the business is quiet? Consider when you are at your freshest or can concentrate best and adjust your daily or weekly plan on that basis. Mindfulness is vital to your role as a leader. Ensure you are present when you work.

Set clear boundaries and stick to them – Do you need 30 minutes each morning to check your emails and set a daily task list to clear your head and make your day more effective? If so, make sure your team knows not to interrupt you unless something is urgent. Being constantly on call can be counterproductive as it means you can never concentrate on one task at a time.

Take breaks and refuel – No one performs at their best without sufficient rest and refreshment, so don't expect yourself to. If you feel foggy or tired, a breath of fresh air, literally, and a glass of water might be just the brain space you need to clear your head and find the solution to the issue you've been dwelling on for 30 minutes. Put time in your diary for you — put some time in every day to do something for you, even just 10 minutes a day focusing on what makes you happy or what you enjoy — there is more to life than just work.

> *'...One of my worst days...I had a ... suicide... motor vehicle accident (death)... a cot death of a baby... and violent domestic... I didn't have time to process anything...'*

Be present in the moment and try not to multitask – It can be tempting to do two or even three things at once, as you can fall into the trap of thinking you will achieve more. While it may often seem necessary to always be available, doing so can add unnecessary stress and pressure, thereby reducing productivity and quality. Don't hesitate to turn off your phone or close your computer when they're not essential to the task at hand, particularly when dealing with staff or other managers. Actively listening and paying proper attention will enhance your ability to relate to people and concentrate on the best solutions and outcomes.

Take time out – You might feel the need to be working every hour of the day to stay on top of everything, but we all need time away from work. Turning off your computer (and your phone) and taking a break will significantly improve your productivity and also set an example for others in your team to follow suit. Research shows that a mere 15-minute walk a day can reduce stress levels, support our mental health, enhance energy levels, and improve cognitive function.

Reflect, learn, and move on – As a leader, you won't get everything right. Leaders often spend too much time dwelling on past mistakes or contemplating what could have been done better. This habit can distract you from moving forward. Spend time reflecting, learn from your experiences, and understand what you'll do differently next time.

Reach out for help – If you ever find yourself overwhelmed, reach out to others who can help. This could include fellow leaders or colleagues, a coach or mentor, friends, family members, or professional support. Never be afraid to seek the help you need.

Say no – Being in a position of leadership doesn't mean you need to agree to everything. Trying to do too much can lead to less efficient outcomes. Recognise that it's okay to say 'no' and focus on your priorities and the areas that will make the most significant difference to you and your organisation.

Although our wellbeing is often within our control, it's important to remember that health, while complex, can also be approached simply.

Being a leader is a privilege, but the significant responsibility of leadership, especially during challenging times, can take its toll on wellbeing and energy levels, leading to feelings of being overwhelmed and potential burnout.

As leaders, we often feel we need to be everything to everyone, but we are all human, and taking care of ourselves should be a priority. By investing in your wellbeing, you become the best version of yourself. You will be healthier and happier, and you will also inspire those around you to do the same. Being an outstanding leader involves looking after others and enabling them to be at their best, which means motivating, inspiring, building trust, being decisive, and making difficult decisions.

Focusing on ourselves might seem a bit egocentric and self-centred, but doing so will help create that balance in life many of us crave. Always ensure that, no matter what happens, you try to prioritise your needs and maintain your self-worth above that of others. By doing so, you will not only be at your best, but also be able to support your family, work colleagues, and friends.

✧

Chapter 15

Leadership in Law Enforcement is A Family Commitment

'Alone, we can do so little; together, we can do so much.'
— Helen Keller

The nature of law enforcement work presents unique challenges that can add stress to an officer's personal relationships, including marriages. Officers encounter distinct hurdles due to their profession, lifestyle, and the inherent culture of their work.

Often, officers work long hours, are exposed to dangerous situations, and witness traumatic events, all of which can take a significant emotional toll. You may also be required to work unconventional schedules, differing from those of their families, making it challenging to spend quality time together. Exposure to organisational injustices can further impact their mental health. These factors can result in a split commitment between work and family roles, perceived personality changes, and can cause officers to carry work-related stress into their home life, leading to difficulties in familial relationships[24].

---

24 https://journals.sagepub.com/doi/pdf/10.1177/1066480714564381

Such pressures can induce feelings of isolation, as sharing their experiences with those outside of the profession can be challenging. The law enforcement culture, often hierarchical and competitive, may further contribute to feelings of alienation from peers and superiors. Moreover, maintaining professional distance from the community you serve, a necessity for your own protection and that of your colleagues, can impede the formation of meaningful personal relationships.

Society is frequently exposed to mass media's portrayal of law enforcement, whether through movies, TV shows, news reports, or social media commentary. These dramatised depictions often become the only frames of reference for many in the general public, skewing perceptions of the challenges faced by law enforcement officers and their families. While some have a more nuanced view of 'law enforcement life' based on personal relationships or past experiences, most lack a realistic basis for their interpretations.

The impact of law enforcement work extends beyond officers themselves. Spouses, partners, parents, children, and other loved ones play a crucial role in an officer's health and wellness, and they too have unique needs[25].

The effects of a law enforcement officer's career are most palpably felt at home. Long hours, rotating shifts, and cancelled leave are realities of law enforcement work. Balancing the demands of a law enforcement career with parental responsibilities often leads officers to miss significant family milestones such as birthdays and school activities.

For many years, there was a marked reluctance within the law enforcement community to recognise the potential

---

25 https://www.theiacp.org/news/blog-post/engaging-families-for-recruitment-and-retention

detrimental effects work on officers' wellbeing, health, and functioning. This hesitation also meant that the impact and stressors of the 'job' on family and loved ones were often overlooked.

The phrase 'canary in a coal mine' serves as a metaphor for an early warning of impending danger. The term originates from the practice of miners carrying caged canaries with them; if the mine contained hazardous gases like methane or carbon monoxide, the canary would succumb before gas levels became lethal to humans, prompting immediate evacuation. My use of this metaphor stems from personal experiences and conversations with other law enforcement officers dealing with mental health issues. Often, it is their loved ones who first notice early signs of declining mental health.

'...I had just been promoted and found myself working sixteen hours a day, as well as most weekends. My wife and children were unhappy. I was scarcely at home, and even when I was, the phone was always ringing. I tried to be a good family man, but it felt impossible. One day, I came home to find they had left, and I was alone. I began drinking heavily. I didn't have anyone to confide in. I requested some time off but was denied, given that I had only just been promoted. The loneliness led to depression. I'm still struggling with depression and feel isolated, yet I can't share this with anyone... '

However, many people are not equipped to identify signs of a problem, especially if their family member is reluctant to open up about their struggles. Therefore, it's crucial for families to be vigilant for early signs, especially if a member is encountering mental health issues for the first time.

A significant concern for an officer is deciding what to share with their family. Avoiding discussions about a particularly challenging day may be the chosen approach. Even if the officer refrains from discussing incidents like fatalities, injured children, vehicle accidents, or organisational injustices, their voice and body language often convey part of the story. The tension between what an officer withholds and what their loved ones wish to understand is a delicate negotiation of boundaries, warranting necessary dialogue.

Being in a relationship with a law enforcement officer certainly presents challenges, but how does this extended exposure to indirect stress and trauma affect their children?

Research has shown that the children of law enforcement officers can vicariously develop traumatic stress through witnessing and listening to their parents. Children may share the same memories or re-enact the officer's trauma, knowing that their parent has experienced such events.

Given the abundance of law enforcement television shows, violent law enforcement/criminal video games, and news stories discussing the job's dangers, it's understandable that law enforcement children may worry about their parents' safety. Signs of anxiety in a child when the law enforcement parent is preparing for work suggest the child is experiencing stress.

While discussing future careers with my 11-year-old daughter, I suggested she could become a police officer like her father. Her response was, 'Why would I do that and end up with PTSD?'

Parents equipped with stress management techniques are less likely to transmit these symptoms to their children as they recognise their own stress responses. Not all children will manifest or internalise their parents' stress. Still, it's something to be mindful of, particularly after a law enforcement parent experiences a traumatic event.

Open communication with your child can help alleviate the stress of the unknown. Fear for a parent's safety will inevitably affect a law enforcement child at some stage.

Reassurances often provide the stress relief that a younger child needs. If your children are older, discuss the job's realities, your training, and safety equipment such as your vest. Sometimes an open dialogue with your teenager is the best way to help them process fear and stress.

While the stress an officer experiences often cannot be altered, some measures can mitigate its impact on their personal life.

- Partner Support: Partners need to comprehend the stressors officers encounter while on duty. By deepening their understanding through education and communication, partners can offer better support to their loved ones. They can also encourage officers to share as much or as little about their job as they feel comfortable.
- Support from Family and Friends: A support network can be an invaluable resource for law enforcement families. Even simple gestures like offering childcare for an evening, allowing an officer and their partner to have some alone time, can be extremely beneficial. Due to the officer's long working hours and shift work, alone time with their partner is often neglected, yet it's a vital aspect of strengthening law enforcement families.
- Socialising with other law enforcement couples or friends can be beneficial. It can be helpful to connect with others who are familiar with the unique challenges of leading a law enforcement family's life.
- Law enforcement officers should strive to maintain an identity separate from their professional role when off-duty. This can be achieved by cultivating hobbies or participating in

activities unrelated to law enforcement. Having a distinct life and identity outside the job helps officers alleviate the pressure of constantly feeling 'on duty'.

- While having connections with other law enforcement families is beneficial, it's equally vital to maintain friendships with couples not involved in law enforcement and those working in different professions. This strategy proves advantageous as both officers and their partners can learn conflict resolution strategies and life perspectives that diverge from the law enforcement mindset.

- Law enforcement departments also play a critical role in supporting their officers' personal relationships. While agencies have provided the necessary engagement and support to families and loved ones, it's important to emphasise the officers' home life support. This can be facilitated by offering engagement programs that educate and incorporate families into the organisational 'fold'. Granting access to dedicated family support services, contact points for concerned family members to reach out to, and assuring family members that reaching out will not adversely impact their partners' standing in the department, is vital.

Chapter 16

The Life Saver —
My Wife's Story

'I have put you through hell and back, but you have unconditionally loved me, my imperfections and flaws. You are so dear to my heart. When I look at you, I fall in love with you all over again.'

— Author to his wife

As we've just explored, maintaining balance in law enforcement duties within a marriage or relationship can present significant challenges.

Below is an unedited, raw, and emotional excerpt from my wife Kate's diary, written during a particularly difficult period in our lives. Kate, who prefers to be referred to as Lordy, penned these words while I was at my worst. Reading it is still tough for me, but I admire her strength, not just for writing it, but also for holding our family together and persevering in supporting me, particularly when I was hard to be around.

> *For so long I felt like I was drowning. But if I drowned, my family would fall apart. I couldn't drown. Hold it together, I would tell myself. I don't have time to drown. Sad. Angry. Exhausted. Scared. Desperate. Isolated. Alone. Guilty.*

That's how I felt living with my husband who had depression, anxiety, and PTSD.

It angered me. Angered me so much that Grant could get up and perform at work every day. Get up and go to training every day. Engage in conversation with work colleagues but not engage with our daughter or myself. Get up and compete in sporting events most weekends. Always find time in his schedule if it was for a doctor's appointment, massage, physio, competitions. But any time outside of these things he slept, or he sat on the couch watching documentaries on the war in Afghanistan. I despised the fact he was doing all his sport while I could do none of mine. I couldn't join a team. I couldn't leave our daughter with him at night while I competed. I didn't trust he wouldn't have taken sleeping pills, drunk bourbon and not hear our daughter if she woke up. He didn't have any spare time or energy left for us. The ones who should have meant the most to him and yet it felt like we meant the least.

Guilt. Terrible guilt that I was so angry with him and yet I knew he was so mentally unwell. What was wrong with me? How selfish was I being? I am strong and capable, and I am angry at my husband while he is sick. It was a vicious cycle for me.

Exhausted. I always was a little OCD but during this time I mastered it. I would wake up a few times every night and check the pool gate. Why? Because Grant would forget to close it properly and then I started having dreams where Jacinta would drown. I would check all the doors were locked as he would often walk outside and then not lock the door behind him. I was scared Jacinta would open the doors and wander out during the night. Paranoia had set in for me. I would vacuum the floors three times a day.

Why? Because Grant was taking so many pills (antihistamine, anti-inflammatory, sleeping pills to name a few) and he would drop them and leave them on the floor. Our daughter was only three. He had boxes of pills everywhere. Briefcase, suitcase, gym bag, throwing bag, bum bag. He would come home with a different bag and leave the bag open, thrown somewhere on the floor. Each time he returned, I would madly look for where he left the bag and pick it up as I was worried our daughter might find the pills in his bag. I couldn't leave our daughter at home with him. Why? Because he would either fall asleep or be so focused on the documentary about Afghanistan, he wouldn't watch her. I would get a phone call from neighbours asking if she was meant to be at their house. Or I would drive up to the house and she would be playing in our front yard near the road unsupervised. I thought if I did everything required for our family (shopping, cooking, cleaning, mowing, gardening, ironing, accounts, managed our properties, raise our daughter, attending all events, etc, etc) during the week, it would free up our weekends so we could do things together as a family. I was wrong and I was exhausted.

I was desperate and alone. I asked his closest friends – How's Grant seem to you? Has he said anything to you? Of course, they all said he was great. He showed them and told them every day at work he was great. I was screaming for help for about two years but couldn't get any. Why? Because he didn't want anyone at work to know and I felt he would hate me even more if he found out I told someone about his current state of mind. I would hint to my friends there was a problem. All of them in short told me how lucky I was. They all thought I had it all. I didn't have to work. I lived in a beautiful home, in a beautiful city with an incredible husband and adorable daughter. All of that is true. But we were falling apart behind closed doors. Some days I couldn't breathe. I would put Jacinta in the car and just drive away from Grant and our home. I'd sit watching the ocean wishing it would all just go away. When I got myself together, I would drive home again.

I was scared. Scared he wanted to leave Jacinta and I. Scared he wasn't in love with me anymore. I didn't make him happy. Jacinta and I weren't enough for him. He wanted so little to do with Jacinta, I would try to fill the gap for her. He was happy training. He was happy competing. He wasn't happy at work as it wasn't as exciting as Afghanistan. This hurt like hell as he felt sorry for himself that he was only watching planes take off and land. In short, I hated his selfishness. He put us through hell while he was in Afghanistan, and we were living a different hell since he returned. But he was 'bored' and I was angry. He was interested in researching all of his medical issues and discussing them with every medical expert he could find. But he was never happy at home with Jacinta and I. It appeared I was a large part of the problem for him. I didn't want to give him any specific reasons to leave me. Having one of his colleagues specifically mention my thoughts/concerns/feelings to him...I thought might just tip him over the edge and he would leave. I couldn't risk it. I focused so hard all the time on making sure he could see I was doing everything for him, and our family was going to be ok.

Grant thought by changing his work location this would improve his life. So he applied for London and got Washington DC.

Moving forward.

Some days I could not be prouder of Grant for the journey he has been on and how far he has come. He is the love of my life, and he is finally content and happy with life. Our family made it. We made it through the other side, and I know without a doubt our family is solid. We will be together for the rest of our lives. But now, instead of surviving through depression I am now supporting someone who has survived depression.

This is when I feel really guilty and selfish again. Now, I feel guilty and angry because I still haven't returned to my old self. I still can't play sports but not because I don't trust Grant to be on his game with our daughter...his work commitments means he is never home. I don't know myself anymore. My old self was always bubbly, laughing, my life was working, training, loved sport and competition. Now I am a glass half-empty person. It's not who I am and it's not who I will always be. I know once we are back in Australia, I will gain my old life back again. But for now, my effort has just shifted from survival to continual support, encouragement and congratulations for all Grant has achieved to ensure we don't return to where we were. I get it. I know what he has achieved is remarkable and deserves every bit of acknowledgement, congratulations, and recognition. The people who aren't acknowledged, congratulated and recognised is US, Jacinta and I. The people who felt – Sad. Angry. Exhausted. Scared. Desperate. Isolated. Alone. Guilty. The family members who didn't have depression, anxiety, and PTS but are living with someone who does.

Jacinta and I survived, too. We were in the same storm, suffering in a different way, but no one is encouraging us or congratulating us for our survival and achievements.

✧

Chapter 17

A New Mindset of Leadership Thinking

*'We cannot solve our problems with the same thinking
we used when we created them.'*

— Albert Einstein

So far, we have examined ways in which you, as a leader, can take care of yourself so that you can be the best version of yourself, leading with energy, confidence, and assurance. A fresh approach to leadership is necessary to address the myriad challenges we face in today's world. The traditional hierarchical model of leadership no longer suffices to handle the complexity and interconnectedness of global issues. We require leaders who can think critically, empathise with others, and collaborate with diverse stakeholders to devise innovative solutions. A new mindset for leadership must also prioritise sustainability and ethical decision-making while recognising the significance of diversity in creating a more equitable society. By shifting our attention from personal gain to collective advantage, we can build a more resilient and equitable future.

The world is increasingly confronting numerous challenges, and there is a growing global desire for change. It's widely accepted that complexity and chaos are indispensable partners in our constantly evolving global environment, especially within law enforcement.

In the ever-evolving VUCA (volatility, uncertainty, complexity, and ambiguity) global environment, leadership challenges present themselves regularly, many with potentially disastrous implications. What is true today may no longer hold tomorrow. More than ever, we live with a lack of predictability and a constant possibility of surprise. Old certainties have evaporated into a haze of grey areas and misunderstandings. We can no longer think in binary terms in a complex world. The profusion of available information has created a fog where clarity becomes increasingly elusive.

Twenty-first century law enforcement leaders must manage swift change and ambiguity in a nonlinear, multidisciplinary, and networked environment. Yet, for the most part, the profession finds itself caught in a process that relies on a paradigm of certainty and predictability. Being an effective leader in this environment requires comfort with operating on the edge of chaos.

Expectations for law enforcement are increasing exponentially at a rapid pace. They are expected to be efficient and effective in an increasingly complex global, social, cultural, and economic environment, whilst remaining ethical and encouraging diverse thinking. They must model inclusivity and respect, demonstrating emotional intelligence and cultural sensitivity. They are required to exercise effective strategic judgement and decision-making, applying critical thinking and problem-solving skills to influence practice, policy, and governance innovatively and creatively[26].

---

26 https://www.utas.edu.au/courses/cale/units/hsp406-police-leadership,-strategy,-and-engagement

The magnitude of the threats currently facing law enforcement indicates that, now more than ever, a highly flexible and agile approach is required, one which involves 'looking outside in, as well as inside out'. In order to respond to the relentlessly volatile landscape that the profession currently faces, agility is crucial. Agility is the capacity to respond quickly and positively to rapid change.

Effective leadership is crucial to organisational success. Many have strived to understand the essence of leadership success for decades, if not centuries. The normative approach to leadership has centred on how leaders must lead from within their organisation. Traditionally, law enforcement organisations have centred their leadership development on strict chains of command, and matrix-type capability where leaders operate across more than one reporting line, usually across functional or business teams. But this outdated model is no longer fit for purpose.

Traditional leadership frameworks are founded on linear thinking, hierarchical structures, rigid top-down controls, imposed plans and solutions, and an excessive focus on efficiency. As a result, leaders cannot simply iterate, recalibrate, reconfigure, or reorganise their way to prosperity. Future-proofing law enforcement leadership requires new thinking, metaphors, assumptions, and values to lead during dynamic and chaotic times. Leaders must introduce new strategies for increasing engagement and motivation, developing emotional and spiritual intelligence so that all members of the institution are empowered to think and act in ways that transcend themselves and their institutions[27]. In short, the leadership methods that got us here won't get us where we need to be.

---

27 https://er.educause.edu/articles/2021/10/the-cio-as-quantum-leader

Trust in law enforcement institutions has been steadily declining recently. At the same time, the profession is grappling with dwindling ranks, plummeting morale, and diminishing public support. The excessive politicisation of law enforcement hasn't helped either.

Senior law enforcement leaders hold a significant position of influence within their organisations. Their roles require balancing fundamental and often conflicting values in environments that are as volatile as any in the competitive global professional landscape.

This has been demonstrated through the recent seismic shift in how organisational middle leaders conduct their work. As cost pressures continue to rise, the demands of governments and elected officials to achieve more with less escalate, and the preference for workers to experience a hybrid work environment reshapes the workplace. Alongside new artificial intelligence and automation technologies, some analysts predict that organisations will need fewer people for traditional middle leadership tasks such as overseeing daily operations, administrative responsibilities, and approving operational workflows.

'I worked in Customs. We received a report of a boat that had sunk while smuggling people into my country. When we finally arrived, all I could see were bodies floating everywhere — women, men, children, even babies. We had to retrieve the bodies. Some had begun to lose their skin. At one point, I was physically sick. My boss yelled at me, saying the bodies were just meat, and told me to toughen up.'

An alternative perspective proposes that in the contemporary hybrid workplace, the importance of middle leaders will magnify.

They will serve as the glue binding teams together, fostering a sense of belonging within organisations. Middle leaders will maintain a pivotal role in the future workplaces, but there will be an increasing demand for the expansion of their capabilities and career trajectories.

It is vital to deviate from the traditional perception of leaders and managers as overseers. Middle leaders play an instrumental role in cultivating talent, fortifying team dynamics, and aiding teams in achieving their objectives.

The advent of technology and automation enables leaders to resolve many issues previously under the purview of middle leaders. This includes dismantling departmental silos, fostering connections between individuals, and expediting processes through workflows and automation. If utilised effectively, these tools negate the necessity for middle leaders to manually monitor aspects like punctuality or project status, freeing them to shift focus from overseeing inputs to strategising on outcomes.

Consequently, progressive departments are increasingly reliant on middle leaders to provide coaching and mentorship, enhance trust, diversity and inclusivity, align team objectives with the broader organisational vision, and inspire innovative ideas for more effective collaboration. Essentially, we are transitioning towards reshaping the role of leaders as facilitators who can coach and develop their teams, as this is what employees genuinely seek and what organisations require to flourish.

As mentioned, outdated mindsets like compelling the younger workforce to conform to existing organisational models and culture are no longer sufficient. Why? Time has proven that a leadership style that resonates with one generation may not engage another as effectively.

The generational composition of the workforce is undergoing significant shifts. By 2025, millennials are projected to constitute 75% of the global workforce. Characteristically, they are civic-minded, accepting of diversity, achievement-oriented, and they seek challenges, growth, personal development, a vibrant work environment and a balanced work-life. Importantly, they are likely to leave an organisation if dissatisfied with a workplace adverse to change. They prefer leaders who take a personal interest in them, manage by results, offer flexibility in schedules and assignments, and provide immediate feedback.

Hot on their heels is Generation Z, now entering the workforce. They are global, entrepreneurial, progressive, and driven by diversity, personalisation, individuality, and creativity. Their communication style leans towards instant messaging, texts, and social media. Often dubbed digital device addicts, they value independence and individuality, prefer to work with millennial managers, innovative colleagues, and emerging technologies[28].

If law enforcement fails to adapt their profession to accommodate new thought paradigms, the influx of new generations, and the evolving world order, then society will impose change. The resulting trajectory may well be beyond their influence and direction.

---

28 https://www.purdueglobal.edu/education-partnerships/generational-workforce-differences-infographic/

✧

Chapter 18

Leadership – Building A Mentally Safe Culture

'You don't have to be positive all the time. It's perfectly okay to feel sad, angry, annoyed, frustrated, scared, and anxious. Having feelings doesn't make you a negative person. It makes you human.'

— Lori Deschene

A mentally safe workplace culture is one where employees feel comfortable discussing mental health issues and are assured of support from their employer in managing these concerns. Such a culture also allows employees to be themselves, free from the fear of discrimination or retaliation.

Creating a mentally safe workplace culture can be achieved through several strategies. Employers can provide access to mental health resources, such as an employee assistance programme or mental health provider. A culture of open communication can be fostered, where employees are encouraged to openly discuss mental health issues without fear of stigma. Moreover, employers can offer training on mental health topics like stress management, or how to recognise and support colleagues who may be struggling with mental health issues.

Culture, a powerful tool that shapes healthy habits, in the context of law enforcement, is broadly defined as the shared norms, values and beliefs of a group. It influences how law enforcement officers perceive their world and their role within it. The attitudes and beliefs they hold about their work, whether as individuals or collectively, directly affect their discretion, decisions, and behaviour. However, the law enforcement culture could be a major obstacle in maintaining psychological health, as it values strength, fearlessness, integrity, stoicism, distrust, self-reliance, controlled demeanour, and emotional resilience. These values can deter help-seeking behaviour and generate a sense of lost control when dealing with a mental health issue. An officer adhering rigidly to these traditional values may feel weak, embarrassed, or like a failure when seeking help, potentially leading to detrimental health effects even when distressed[29].

Factors such as stress, heavy workloads, poor communication, uncertainty, and other elements can all contribute to anxiety and depression. Leaders have the responsibility to manage these factors. They should prioritise mental health as an organisational goal, with clear ownership and accountability mechanisms, rather than relegating it to HR. Leaders can foster transparency and openness by sharing their personal experiences, thereby acting as allies. Without a stigma-free culture, even organisations with superior mental health benefits may not see an increase in their use due to fear and shame.

To make this effective, organisations need to train leaders, managers, and all employees on handling mental health at work, conducting difficult conversations, and creating supportive workplaces. Managers, often the first to notice changes and provide

29 http://www.policechiefmagazine.org/magazine/index.cfm?fuseaction=display&
   article_id=3354&issue_id=52014

support to their direct reports, play a crucial role. Establishing an environment of psychological safety is key. Implementing and over-communicating about mental health policies, culturally competent benefits, and other resources is essential.

While the voice of senior management is crucial and influential, employees at every level can also significantly influence how mental health is addressed in the workplace. Successful mental health support efforts must reach and educate all employees, integrating these into the daily workplace environment. This inclusive approach effectively combats stigma, fosters widespread awareness among all employees about the importance of mental health, regardless of their personal situation.

'...I worked in a job where a senior executive of a government department was alleged to have interfered with children. My boss wanted me to arrest and charge him. There was evidence that the executive did what was alleged, but it occurred in another country, and that country did not have a law that could be used. Although I wanted to arrest him, the deficiency in the law would not allow me to do so. My boss was angry, berated me in front of my colleagues, and I was placed on report for being lazy. It hurt me deeply. Eventually, I was proven right, but there was no apology, nor did my boss withdraw the report...'

When leadership fails to seize the opportunity to collaborate, listen, and empathise, trust, commitment, and engagement are lost. The consequence is that the responsibility of advancing better mental health retreats into 'bunker' mode. Good ideas and honest dialogue are dismissed, allowing the existing model to persist. This indifference effectively stifles all prospects of growth, collaboration, and engagement.

I've encountered toxic work culture firsthand, replete with its many negatives. The hallmarks were easy to spot; one need only assess the quality, or lack thereof, of the leadership team. Capable leaders inspire high levels of trust, engagement, and productivity, while incompetent ones foster anxiety and alienation, leading to counterproductive behaviours and a spread of toxicity throughout the organisation.

The influence of law enforcement culture on mental health can be profound. Law enforcement often forms a microcosm in which a close-knit society perpetuates a code of silence, secretive behaviour, and a mutual reliance for survival. It embodies a set of assumptions, beliefs, expectations, and philosophies that govern professional interactions, performance, and roles. This culture informs law enforcement officers on their approach to tasks, work intensity, relationship dynamics with fellow officers and other individuals they interact with, and their attitudes towards law enforcement executives, judges, laws, and the mandates they impose.

For a law enforcement officer, the act of asking someone else for help, especially in the face of public expectations of unflappability, can feel like an egregious loss of control. These cultural norms discourage help-seeking behaviours and inhibit potential disclosure of mental health issues. An officer might easily request leave for a physical illness like a migraine or flu, but discussing mental health conditions can be a significant hurdle. Officers may hesitate to broach the subject with family, friends, and colleagues, let alone their superiors. Acknowledging a mental health condition within the law enforcement culture is often seen as a sign of weakness, a potential career ender, and a label that could lead to discrimination, isolation, and alienation. Fearful of being perceived as weak, untrustworthy, or risking sanctions and professional setbacks, officers are often reluctant to seek help, even privately.

Incompetent leaders are a primary cause of low employee engagement, presenteeism, high discontent levels, and passive workplace practices. Over the years, I've observed that employees who distrust their managers and leadership teams often cite similar concerns: unethical behaviour, concealment of information, taking undue credit, or outright deception. I've seen untrustworthy managers sap morale, hinder productivity, unduly stress their staff, and, in some cases, ruin careers. If employees remain tight-lipped about their concerns until their manager leaves the room, only then voicing grievances about secrecy, bullying, and a tendency to set staff members against one another, the issues are apparent.

Transitioning from distrust to trust can yield substantial personal and organisational benefits, such as increased information exchange, leading to enhanced leadership effectiveness and efficiency. Yet, distrust is pervasive in law enforcement, worldwide, across all types of departments and organisations. Although trust is at an all-time low, there are strategies available to enhance your leadership trust factor.

Determine your employees' needs

Consult with your organisation and staff to assess your workplace's mindset and practices concerning mental health. What improvements could be made? What existing strategies are effective?

Identify risk factors that can negatively impact mental health. Some of these include:

• Long work hours over extended periods
• Heavy workloads

- Unrealistic deadlines
- Insufficient support
- Unclear role definitions and success measures
- Lack of recognition at work
- Toxic workplaces where bullying or discrimination occurs

Support your staff in managing workloads — be flexible

Assisting people in managing their workload also involves listening to employees and understanding common stress triggers.

Exercise caution with heavy workloads, set realistic deadlines, and manage uncertainty. Identify areas with inadequate support, especially for new hires. If they lack mentors or supportive bosses, it becomes a risk factor. Prioritise workloads and plan jobs in collaboration with staff.

I've often found that giving people autonomy over their work methods, timings, and interactions with others can significantly impact both the individual and the organisation. It provides them a greater sense of control over their work life and helps them stay mindful of their mental health needs.

Establish a psychologically safe culture

Creating a psychologically safe work culture can enhance retention efforts by fostering a sense of belonging. In such an environment, employees feel empowered to voice their concerns, feel valued, and receive support from managers and co-workers. It's crucial for managers to stay aware of staff well-being consistently, not only when employees are unwell.

In a psychologically unsafe workplace, employees remain silent when they should voice concerns. They fear consequences for speaking up and believe that new ideas will face criticism.

Taking a mental health day

Mental health days are paid or unpaid days off that employees can utilise to focus on their well-being. Although they can be used for various reasons, the main goal is to support an employee's productivity and retention by encouraging self-care. Both employees and employers can benefit from mental health days, but many people seldom utilise them. This article provides tips on how to take a mental health day without feeling guilty.

Despite mental health becoming a more prevalent topic of discussion, many individuals still hesitate to discuss mental health days with their managers or colleagues. This is usually due to workplace culture and the stigma attached to mental health issues in the community.

On numerous occasions, I've had to take a day or two off work for my mental health. However, most of the time, I'd fabricate a physical ailment like gastro or a cold when calling in sick. Sadly, many people I've discussed this with also resort to fabricating physical illnesses to avoid potential backlash from declaring a mental health day.

Promoting open communication, respect, diversity, and inclusion, along with fostering team connectedness, relationships, and celebrating achievements, contribute to creating a supportive and constructive workplace culture.

Prioritise support and communication every day

Creating a mentally healthy workplace requires more than sporadic resilience training sessions. It's a long-term commitment that involves cultivating an environment where employees feel consistently safe and supported, and mental health is openly discussed.

The days of not addressing mental health should be over. Positive mental health is important as it enables individuals to manage challenges and setbacks in their lives, both at work and at home.

Positive mental health at work assists teams in staying agile during role and responsibility changes, as well as while facing difficult challenges. It enables employees to thrive in their roles, manage stress, and enhance resilience. In essence, it empowers everyone to reach their highest potential.

Creating a safe space for employees at all levels to communicate openly without discrimination is crucial. Without this, you risk missing out on valuable feedback that could help retain talent.

Even if an organisation offers excellent mental health programs and training, these resources will be ineffectual unless employees feel safe discussing their issues without fearing negative consequences.

If an employee is returning to work after a mental health absence, have a supportive plan in place, such as flexible sick leave and workload adjustments. Sometimes, returning to work can be grounding and comforting for those who have experienced a mental health issue.

Furthermore, it's essential to maintain a zero-tolerance policy towards bullying and discrimination.

Sadly, I have often been taken aback by how often toxic workplaces with bullying, sexism, racism, or harassment are overlooked by senior management. Leaders must set a positive tone in the workplace, which includes not tolerating or enabling negative behaviour.

Benefits of a psychologically healthy workplace

As an employer, you have various methods to foster a psychologically healthy and safe workplace. Creating a supportive environment that promotes mental well-being benefits everyone and ensures your workforce remains robust and competitive. Advantages include heightened engagement, increased morale, work satisfaction, improved retention and recruitment, and boosted productivity. Other benefits include reduced absentee- ism and grievances, lowered health costs and insurance premi- ums, and fewer workplace injuries.

Establishing a mentally safe workplace culture is crucial for several reasons. Firstly, employees who feel mentally safe at work are more likely to be productive and engaged. Additionally, men- tally safe workplaces are associated with lower absenteeism and staff turnover. Finally, employees who feel mentally safe are more likely to voice concerns or problems, helping prevent accidents or incidents in the workplace.

Chapter 19

Investment Rather Than Reaction

'If you can't fly, run. If you can't run, walk.
If you can't walk, crawl, but by all means, keep moving.'
— Martin Luther King, Jr.

As we've seen, numerous factors contribute to mental health and well-being, and workplace mental health is a crucial issue that's garnered increasing attention in recent years.

Several reasons contribute to the lack of financial investment in law enforcement. Governments often hesitate to invest in workplace mental health due to fear of the unknown. The issue is so widespread that governments fear the costs associated with supporting the psychologically injured members — through elevated insurance premiums, staff shortages, and potential medical retirement — will significantly impact their budgets. Therefore, ignorance, obfuscation, and plausible deniability are often chosen options.

Additionally, mental health problems can be difficult to identify and diagnose, making it hard to justify expenditure to decision-makers. A lack of awareness of the importance of workplace mental health, and its impact on productivity, safety, and morale, persists. Some governments believe workplace mental health is a personal responsibility, absolving them of the need to address these issues. Finally, some view mental health initiatives as a 'soft' issue and fear investing in such programs will be seen as squandering taxpayer resources.

Despite the challenges surrounding workplace mental health, a growing body of evidence suggests investing in these programs offers numerous benefits. Thus, it's vital for decision-makers to recognise the importance of workplace mental health and con-sider how the government can financially support these programs.

Without suitable funding and support, departmental and organisational heads often need to shuffle priorities to secure funds from existing budgets. This usually results in the creation of a minimal program that serves as a start but is minimally effective.

Investing in mental health directly reflects how an organisation prioritises action on mental health. Research has indeed found positive returns on investment (ROI) from workplace mental health initiatives. Prioritising employee wellbeing is more than an obligation. Organisations that prioritise mental health in the workplace reap numerous benefits, including[30]:

- A positive return on investment. Every dollar spent on men-tal health initiatives, on average, sees a return on investment of $2.50–$4.
- Improved recruitment and retention efforts. By building a positive workplace with happy and healthy staff, your organ-isation can attract and retain the best talent.
- Higher levels of engagement and work performance. Staff members are more likely to be engaged in a positive

---

30 https://www2.deloitte.com/ca/en/pages/press-releases/articles/significant-roi-for-workplace-mental-health-programs.html

work environment. Greater employee engagement leads to improved performance, enhanced work quality, and increased productivity.

- A workplace mental health strategy drives organisational change and promotes a healthy work environment. Whether you're just starting or looking to develop your strategy, these steps can help you build a solid foundation.
- However, it's important to remember that each department and organisation is different, so tailoring a response to your organisation's needs and structure is crucial.

Wellness programs are more likely to achieve a positive ROI when they support employees along the entire spectrum of mental health, from early intervention, education, promotion of well-being, to intervention and ongoing care.

Law enforcement can achieve greater program ROI by prioritising investment in higher-impact areas such as leadership training and preventive interventions, including psychological care benefits.

If departments measure their baseline data and review existing initiatives, many organisations will realise they have already begun using the right tools to strengthen workplace mental health.

Creating a workplace culture that values mental health doesn't need to be a costly endeavour. In many cases, plenty of low-hanging fruit can bear rewards for employers.

Creating a culture of open communication and respect is a good start. This can be done by promoting a culture of openness about mental health, and by supporting employees who are struggling with mental health issues. Simple education programmes aim at designing a healthy workplace environment by promoting healthy lifestyle choices and creating a physically and emotionally safe workplace. They also form appropriate

> *'...I worked in a predominantly female area as a civilian. We got a new supervisor who was horrible. He would tell the most inappropriate jokes and make terrible comments to us. He would even place his penis on a table to call out to us so we would look. The environment was terrible. I made a complaint, but nothing happened; the behaviour didn't change. Instead, I was moved into a back office and made to work alone. I was the one who was punished...'*

human resource processes related to taking leave and returning to work, along with policies that promote mental health and wellbeing.

However, the establishment of a programme, no matter how small or large, funded or not, doesn't end with its implementation. Measurement and evaluation (M&E) are critical in any ongoing initiative that attracts financial allocation. Without M&E, how can you ascertain the effectiveness of a programme or initiative?

'If you can't measure it, you can't improve it.' This famous business maxim, attributed to renowned management and leadership expert Peter Drucker[31], serves an even higher purpose today. Applied to workplace mental health, law enforcement leaders can elevate their initiatives and play a leading role in creating psychologically safe, healthy, and supportive workplaces. This can improve the lives of millions of workers grappling with mental health challenges.

---

31 https://twitter.com/virtualtlc

The value of mental health benefits has long been puzzling for employers. As employee demand rises, the question presents itself: How do we know if it's worth it[32]?

Leaders who prioritise mental health understand the importance of measuring and tracking improvements in programmes. Using metrics not only guides revisions and adjustments that make initiatives more effective, but also sends a powerful signal to employees that achieving mental health goals is as important as hitting revenue targets.

Firstly, departments need to define what 'good' looks like. Many leaders are well-intentioned, but they can't articulate the problem they're trying to solve or the results they hope to achieve. Agencies must clearly define the desired outcome and practise principles of change management to work step-by-step towards that goal, making continuous adjustments along the way.

Secondly, executives need to be accountable for results. The dialogue around mental health and wellbeing is now occurring at the senior executive leadership level. By integrating mental health metrics into frameworks, departments can create a culture of accountability that drives improvements and reassures elected officials and governments that their investments are making a difference and are worthwhile.

Thirdly, agencies need to apply more rigour to their metrics. This can be achieved by continuously measuring improvement, uptake, awareness, and utilisation across various mental health initiatives. Widely used pulse surveys can be helpful, as can employee assistance program utilisation measures, aside from the basic engagement statistics. After all, it's about more than just numbers.

---

32 https://onemind.org/workplace-mental-health-blogs/measuring-progress-on-workplace-mental-health/

Perhaps most importantly, leaders need to understand that merely creating a suite of mental health benefits and hoping employees use them isn't a strategy. By applying such wisdom, executives can start to define the problem, measure progress, and make adjustments that will result in a happier, healthier, more loyal, and more productive workforce.

✦

Chapter 20

One Size Doesn't Fit All

'The shoe that fits one person pinches another;
there is no recipe for living that suits all cases.'

— Karl Jung

Existing institutional governance, policy, and structures relating to mental health within law enforcement are relatively rare. Most departments have not successfully developed or incorporated mental health objectives within their organisational and governance structures.

The creation and execution of clearly defined mental health policies and plans are crucial to good governance and leadership for mental health in law enforcement. These contribute to improving the organisation, accessibility, and quality of service delivery, and fostering engagement with stakeholders. This includes prevention, early intervention, those with lived experience, their families and loved ones, and the broader law enforcement community. Key elements include setting clear targets and areas for action, allocating sufficient resources, using an evidence-based approach, and showing a commitment to support[33].

---

33 http://www.justice.gov/archive/ag/speeches/2005/051605agdeamemorial.htm

Governance is a vital component of any organisation. It's about the time dedicated to working 'on' your organisation, rather than 'in' it. Governance encompasses all practices, processes, and policies guiding your organisation in the right direction, such as developing a mental health program.

Mental health policy and governance in the workplace can be challenging for some organisations due to concerns about employee privacy, confidentiality, and potential impacts on insurance costs. For instance, if an employee becomes suicidal, there's no guarantee they won't act on the impulse. Organisations often protect themselves legally by implementing mental health policies at their workplace, which can lead to the perception that the policy is more about protecting the agency rather than supporting the affected individual.

Establishing a governance structure for mental health demonstrates to staff that the organisation is committed to embedding mental health into its language. Institutions can unintentionally adopt a tokenistic approach to mental health, hosting one-off events such as morning teas for R U Okay? Day or mindfulness classes to address stress. While these events can complement a broader approach, it's no longer viable for single or tokenistic events to constitute the entirety of an organisation's efforts. Organisations need to make mental wellness part of their institutional DNA.

Due to the nature of law enforcement work and the associated culture, officers dealing with personal crises or emotional distress often feel they have no support. This may be due to the stigma attached to admitting the need for help, which could be viewed as a sign of weakness or an indication they are unfit for duty.

Sometimes, these fears are reinforced by official organisational policy, which can lead officers to believe that these policies are solely for organisational protection. Certain agencies require officers seeking or receiving mental health treatment, or those taking psychotropic drugs, to inform the department and possibly face duty restrictions during their treatment. This type of stigma or misunderstanding perpetuates misinformation, trapping law enforcement officers in a cycle of depression, anxiety, or similar situations[34].

Implementing a comprehensive institutional and cultural reshaping program that integrates mental health processes into the organisation can reduce officer scepticism and distrust, fostering a culture that encourages help-seeking behaviour.

Mental health policy can assist by providing services to those suffering from mental illness. However, this is often not the goal for many employers due to the associated costs. Mental health policy can be used for both preventive and intervention purposes, and it also assists workers in returning to work. This is crucial because extended absences can increase costs for employers in health-care bills. Additional benefits of a mental health policy include lower rates of disability claims and improved job performance, as those suffering from mental illnesses often exhibit poorer job performance due to the impact on their mood and energy levels.

'...One of the worst parts of law enforcement is having to do the "death knock"... being the one to inform a loved one that their child, husband, wife, brother, or sister has died... It never gets easier... Each one kind of sits with you... Your body just stores the trauma...'

Mental health policy is crucial for employers as it can reduce absenteeism, tardiness, and workplace turnover, often resulting from mental illness. Employers aim to promote mental health

34 https://www.police1.com/police-products/human-resources/articles/suffering-in-silence-mental-health-and-stigma-in-policing-mjOp9cyzKIPz4jMz/

awareness in the workplace and highlight its benefits. A mental health policy also assists those suffering from mental illness by facilitating their return to work, reducing disability claims, and improving workplace performance. Those suffering from such conditions often face challenges with mood and energy levels.

Promoting mental health awareness through policy is an effective strategy. If employers have programs to support those suffering from mental illness, these employees may feel more motivated and perform better at work, thereby increasing employee commitment and loyalty[35].

In professions where people are frequently exposed to stress, trauma, and human misery, like law enforcement, shaping the institutional environment can help formalise, normalise, and lessen the stigma contributing to the resistance of seeking support and treatment.

Institutional strengthening is an imperative for organisations wishing to develop or enhance existing or new systems. This improvement helps cultivate and retain the skills, knowledge, and resources needed to competently perform their roles and responsibilities in wellbeing. It enables individuals and organisations to perform at a greater capacity.

Institutional strengthening moves organisations beyond short-term implementations and outcomes. It aims to enhance capacity, in this case mental health, within law enforcement communities. This implies a long-term, strategic-level shift towards sustainability in organisational and individual mindsets.

Organisations and leaders who aim to be successful must understand their staff — the target group they seek to mobilise, organise, influence, or recruit. Effectiveness is achieved by learning from these individuals, understanding their conditions, and

---

35 https://mantracare.org/employee-wellness/mental-health-policy/

driving change at a pace they can accept, for example, within law enforcement subcultures[36].

Networking aims to bolster capacity and prevent fragmentation of efforts by promoting collaboration, sharing resources (human, technical, institutional), and fostering a culture of discussion and communication among all affected parties. This necessitates cooperative mechanisms among education and training institutions, as well as public and private sectors.

Partnership arrangements aim to complement efforts by leveraging the strengths and addressing the weaknesses of partners. Major actors in these partnerships might include other law enforcement agencies, universities, the private sector, government, and local communities.

Institutional strengthening requires a systems-thinking approach to performance improvement. While change typically occurs at the individual and organisational level, it is vital to apply these principles to external systems and relationships with key stakeholders, working collectively for change.

With supportive systems in place, an organisation can strategically pursue their mission, adapt to a changing environment, and positively impact the system within which they operate.

Proper governance requires time and thought from committed leaders who understand the benefits of aligning every level of an organisation to produce desired results. Good corporate governance ensures a department's environment is fair and transparent, and that employees can be held accountable for their actions.

Conversely, weak corporate governance leads to waste, mismanagement, and poor integrity. Regardless of the type of venture, only good governance can deliver sustainable and robust business performance.

---

36 https://etu.org.za/toolbox/docs/building/constituency.html

✦

Chapter 21

Building A Mental Health Business Case

*'There still are so many people who are suffering in silence.
And there's still this stigma attached to mental health
which we've got to completely obliterate.'*
— HRH The Duke of Cambridge

The business case for workplace mental health is compelling. Investing in employee mental health can lead to increased productivity, lower health care costs, and improved employee engagement and retention.

The business case presents the problem or opportunity, explores options, analyses costs, benefits, and risks, and ultimately backs a recommendation for an investment decision. The business case should explicitly outline the policy problem the investment aims to address, directly linking to the goals and objectives of the proposed investment[37].

Considered the key document for supporting investment decisions, the business case should be continually updated

---

37 https://www.finance.gov.au/government/commonwealth-investment-framework/
commonwealth-investments-toolkit/developing-business-case

throughout the development and decision-making process. This allows for the inclusion of the most accurate information available, considering whole-of-life cycle implications.

A business case for workplace mental health should be comprehensive and well-structured. It needs to identify the costs associated with mental health issues in the workplace, such as reduced productivity, absenteeism, and turnover, and demonstrate how investing in mental health initiatives can mitigate these costs. It should also outline the potential benefits of investing in mental health initiatives, including increased employee engagement and morale, improved physical health outcomes, and enhanced decision-making. Finally, it should incorporate a clear action plan outlining the proposed initiatives' implementation, along with a timeline.

Studies show that departments improving employee wellbeing performance by 3.5% see a 1% increase in employee satisfaction. Organisations that enhance employee wellbeing performance by 4% see a 1% increase in satisfaction and a 1% decrease in employee turnover. Therefore, focusing on mental health can be key to attracting emerging Generation Z talent, setting them up for success in the workplace.

However, developing a business case for workplace mental health can present challenges. Quantifying the benefits of investing in mental health initiatives can be difficult. Defining the problem, calculating the cost of inaction, and estimating the return on investment pose other challenges.

For a workplace mental health strategy to succeed, those in leadership positions should lead the charge. Stakeholders possess differing values and priorities. Some fully support workplace mental health initiatives, while others may require persuasion. Regardless, securing their commitment is essential before initiating any programs.

To build a strong business case, one of the best starting points is to examine why it's important for your organisation to establish or enhance its mental health strategy. Integrating arguments appealing to the diverse parties involved in your workplace mental health strategy can fortify your case. These arguments can underscore the financial benefits, the ethical importance of workplace mental health, or the impact on your organisation's public image. Support your arguments with statistics about mental health in the workplace and use best practices to demonstrate how successful initiatives benefit organisations and their employees[38].

'...If I'm told one more time by my organisation that I have to be more resilient, I'll cry. Why is it always up to me to try and become more resilient? The organisation doesn't help me; instead, there's just an expectation that I have to figure it out on my own...'

Before implementing new initiatives, it's often helpful to develop a base to work from. The best place to start is by conducting a situational needs analysis to assess existing mental health practices and identify any gaps. Examine your existing policies and procedures, taking into account the following:

- Do you have policies and practices in place to support the wellbeing and mental health of employees?
- Does your organisation meet legal obligations, including work health and safety standards?
- Do employees have a designated place to seek support? Is there an established employee assistance program?
- Is your organisation supportive of flexible work schemes?

---

38 https://www.mybusiness.com.au/how-we-help/be-a-better-employer/managing-people/how-to-develop-workplace-mental-health-strategy

- Do you have a response plan that helps managers and colleagues identify signs of mental illness in the workplace?
- Does your workplace offer mental health training?
- It's also useful to understand how your organisation performs when compared to industry benchmarks. This can include factors such as absenteeism, workers' compensation claims, turnover rates, or workplace productivity reports. An employee survey can reveal valuable insights into any existing issues or attitudes towards workplace mental health.

Going forward, these data can serve as a baseline for measuring your efforts and help identify areas for improvement.

Using the results of your audit, you should have valuable information to inform your action plan.

From the list of issues, firstly identify those that will have the most significant impact on employee mental health and wellbeing. Then, rank the issues based on your organisation's level of motivation to affect change. Those that are most impactful and have the highest level of buy-in from stakeholders should be prioritised in your action plan.

From this, establish three to five clear objectives for your organisation to focus on. These should be divided into short, medium, and long-term actions and KPIs. Regardless of the objective, your goals and outcomes should follow the specific, measurable, achievable, relevant, and timely (S.M.A.R.T.) goal principles.

After setting your goals, identify the resources and expertise needed to achieve them. This might include internal experts or external organisations involved in your jurisdiction.

Feedback and communication are crucial to the success of your workplace mental health strategy. Set regular check-in points to monitor the outcomes of your initiatives against your objectives and KPIs — some refer to these as milestone points. These should be frequent at the start of an initiative to build momentum and raise awareness: for example, once every week or every fort-night. Once teams are on board, you can reduce the frequency to monthly or quarterly.

During these sessions, focus on gathering feedback from dif-ferent elements of the organisation. Evaluate the actions that are effective and celebrate these successes with your team. Additionally, examine any challenges your organisation may be facing, and work together to find actions that may help resolve these.

Developing a solid business case for investment can help build a mentally healthy workplace. With the right case and support from leadership, the success of a business case will contribute to cultivating a positive work culture in your organisation.

At the end of this book, you'll find a series of generalised tem-plates that may help you begin developing your business case for a mental health program in the workplace.

Chapter 22

How Should A Mental Health Program Look?

'When "I" is replaced by "we", even illness becomes wellness.'
— Charles Roppel

Implementing a wellness program is not a 'one-size-fits-all' endeavour. Agencies must tailor their wellness initiatives to meet their specific needs. Law enforcement agencies should proactively promote member wellness through an innovative programming approach, as personal wellness is multifaceted and requires an inclusive and holistic approach. Addressing wellness is not limited to simply improving physical fitness or offering psychological counselling services[39].

What this shows us is that mental health needs to be understood from biological, psychological, as well as sociocultural perspectives, also referred to as the biopsychosocial viewpoint. The biopsychosocial model is an interdisciplinary model that examines the interconnection between biology, psychology, and socio-environmental factors. The model specifically looks at how these aspects play a role in mental health, alongside

---

39 https://link.springer.com/article/10.1057/s41285-018-0065-6

leadership and organisational cultural imperatives to form an integrated ecosystem for mental health in law enforcement.

The Socio-ecological model of mental health reflects the multidirectional complexity and dynamic interplay among factors operating within and across respective levels, from macro (societal) through micro (individual). These factors play out so that environments affect people both personally and corporately while individual and collective actions can conversely impact an immediate or more extended milieu. The model respects the reality that intervention can be made at a variety of points to strengthen resilience and remove or reduce negative features, and that complementary activity on several fronts can yield greater combined benefit than initiatives focused only on one level or area. As such, it calls for interdisciplinary collaborative efforts to adequately address the diversity of issues that bear on the health of a community of people. It thus provides a framework for determining and directing strategies that can together comprise a consistent, coherent response with cumulative force to effect positive change in the law enforcement workplace[40].

In order to prevent mental illness and promote mental health, there is a need to simultaneously target several multilayered factors, not just look at one determinant in isolation like PTSD, suicide, or peer support. The connected and collective elements of mental health need to be amalgamated into a system that considers all the elements previously discussed. That system is a mental health ecosystem.

Mental health ecosystems are a whole-systems approach to mental healthcare, facilitating the analysis of the complex environment and context of mental health systems, and the translation of this knowledge into policy and practice. In law enforcement, the

---

40 https://www.heretohelp.bc.ca/infosheet/promoting-positive-mental-health-through-a-socio-ecological-approach

mental health ecosystem can be seen as a subset of the general health system, which focuses on areas relevant to mental health. For law enforcement, it will focus on characteristics of the profession, the specific elements of the workforce, and the broader organisation responsible for providing care and support to its members, their connections, and the relationships between internal and external stakeholders[41].

The law enforcement mental health ecosystem further relates to the totality of circumstances comprising components, which together provide capital to 'sustain and enhance an organisation's human wellbeing' capacity, including individual capital, social capital, cultural capital, leadership capital and financial capital, all aimed at strengthening the institution to appropriately address their individual organisational needs.

Developing and implementing a wellness program is not a one-size-fits-all endeavour. Merging leadership, culture, institutional strengthening, and biopsychosocial determinants through a socio-ecological model will enhance the understanding of the dynamic interplay between personal and environmental factors within law enforcement, supporting a better organisational mental health approach. The factors and behaviours impacting an officer's mental health are broad, intricate, and diverse. Agencies must tailor their wellness initiatives to meet their distinct social, cultural, and departmental needs through a multifaceted, inclusive, and holistic innovative programming approach. Agency leaders should consider related topics such as promoting individual financial health, improving nutrition, advancing sleep hygiene, and extending support to family and retired members. Of paramount significance is appealing to the hearts and minds of staff, emphasising that their health and well-being is of utmost importance.

---

41 https://www.ncbi.nlm.nih.gov/pmc/articles/PMC8274404/

The goal is to prevent law enforcement officers from incurring a mental health injury in the first place[42].

> *'...Every time I handle a case where a child is assaulted, molested, raped, or abused, I can't help but think about my own kids... I know we're not supposed to personalise things... but we're human, too... it's impossible for me not to do that... it changes the way I parent my children...'*

The socio-ecological framework can be an ideal tool for addressing these broad issues and implementing new mental health programs through integrating behavioural, leadership, and cultural and environmental changes. This model is typically used to explain an approach, program, governance, and policy that will have an impact on greater acceptance and participation in conceptualising an implementable and deliverable strategy. A comprehensive strategic framework should identify and develop agency-specific needs for creating and enhancing a mental health program.

It's difficult at the best of times to change human behaviour, particularly in an environment like law enforcement, which often resists change. The factors and behaviours impacting an officer's mental health are complicated and diverse — no one size fits all (i.e., a vanilla response doesn't work). Therefore, the socio-ecological model is used to provide a sort of charter to help understand the various factors that are enablers or potential barriers to mental health recognition and participation.

All aspects of the socio-ecological framework require simultaneous attention. They are symbiotically reliant on each other's

---

42 https://www.policechiefmagazine.org/the-divergence-of-institution-leadership-culture/

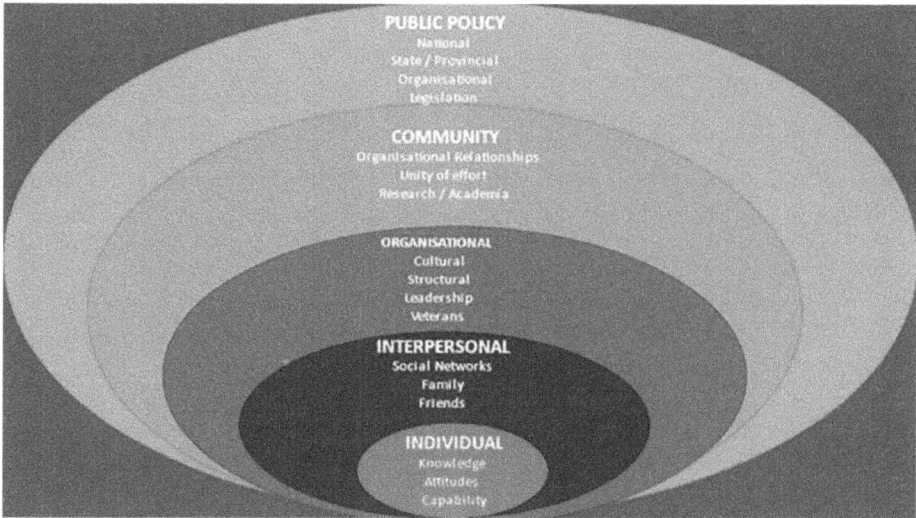

PUBLIC POLICY
National
State / Provincial
Organisational
Legislation

COMMUNITY
Organisational Relationships
Unity of effort
Research / Academia

ORGANISATIONAL
Cultural
Structural
Leadership
Veterans

INTERPERSONAL
Social Networks
Family
Friends

INDIVIDUAL
Knowledge
Attitudes
Capability

growth, such as governments or elected officials' financial and policy support; governance, capability, and organisational relationship enhancement; social and cultural reform; enhanced leadership understanding and training; social connectedness strategies; and individual knowledge and literacy extension. When you fuse leadership, culture, and institutional strengthening into a socio-ecological model, you have a comprehensive strategic schematic to identify and develop agency-specific needs for creating or enhancing a mental health framework. However, success requires change!

More effort needs to be directed towards not only the behaviour choices of individuals, but also towards the aspects that shape those choices to increase greater mental health resilience. Research suggests that the social, physical, and policy environments, when used concurrently, can all influence the ability or likelihood of individuals engaging in a better mental health program. Therefore, the socio-ecological model is important, as it can help to classify possibilities to promote trust, support, and participation by recognising multiple significant factors influencing a person's individual behaviour.

In the context of law enforcement, such a model is typically used to explain an approach, program, and policy that will have an impact on greater acceptance and participation in conceptualising a program. They can be used to understand specific issues in a certain situation or context. One way it can be used is by pinpointing and identifying factors related to poor mental health in specific sectors, enabling a suite of actions in developing an appropriate plan for an effective strategy.

First-tier leaders need to be proactive in gathering the facts, particularly regarding policies like self-isolation and how it's managed in reality. As frontline staff, leaders must remember that they're not just dealing with their own emotions and those of their friends and family members. They're also dealing with a wide range of consistent emotional responses from others. That's a lot of emotion!

Every aspect of the socio-ecological framework needs to be addressed simultaneously – they each depend on the growth of one another. That encompasses government/elected official support, governance, capability, organisational relationships, cultural reform, elevated leadership understanding and training, social connectedness, and individual knowledge growth, capability and attitudes.

✧

Chapter 23

Why Should We Care About Protecting Our Protectors?

Even at times it feels like the whole world is throwing bricks at you,
it's important that you be supported and protected

— author

I n summary, there are several reasons why we should care about protecting our protectors. Firstly, they keep us safe. These individuals put their lives on the line daily to shield us from harm. Their dedication allows us to sleep soundly at night, reassured of our safety.

Secondly, they deserve our respect. They've chosen a job that's often thankless and hazardous. They aren't in it for glory or money. They're driven by a belief in something greater than themselves. They believe in our safety, justice, and our right to live peacefully.

Thirdly, we must remember that they are human beings, just like us. They have families and loved ones who worry about them constantly. They harbour hopes and dreams like ours. They merit our support and care.

We've acknowledged the challenges law enforcement faces regularly, both inside and outside their departments, and how these can impact their health, wellbeing, and mental health. Attempts to mitigate the job's effects, though commendable, have focused on reducing suicide rates and addressing wellbeing and mental health through the lens of social determinants, using the biopsychosocial model of healthcare.

Unfortunately, without leadership at all levels of law enforcement, these initiatives struggle to gain traction and hence lack sustainability. Leadership is the critical element that, until now, has been absent in ensuring a program's success within a department.

In this book, I've endeavoured to highlight the urgent need to develop specific capabilities and capacities in mental health leadership, particularly in law enforcement workplaces. The data speaks for itself: the profession struggles with high levels of mental health injuries and suicide. Law enforcement departments, though well-intentioned, are missing a crucial component to ensure a comprehensive, effective, and manageable support mechanism for their staff.

The current lack of evidence-based research and adequate data and information on law enforcement mental health leadership is minimal, underscoring the necessity for education and training in developing leaders' capabilities in mental health leadership skills.

In the introduction, I promised to share my insight, experience, training qualifications, and thoughts on why it's so important that leaders develop mental health capabilities in the workplace. So, here's a summary of everything I've shared to educate, guide, and provide a new suite of skills that will enhance how law enforcement professionals lead their staff with a sound mental health capacity. It includes:

- Identifying why law enforcement is in the midst of a global mental-health crisis.

- Offering suggestions on how to improve your own health and wellbeing.
- Developing an understanding of common mental health issues and their possible functional impacts.
- Learning how to recognise symptoms and respond to mental health issues in the workplace.
- Acquiring skills to fulfil your workplace responsibilities on mental health.
- Developing strategies to discuss mental health and performance concerns with employees.
- Designing reasonable workplace adjustments for employees with mental health conditions.
- Understanding the impact on your family, typically passive participants, on the effects the job has on their loved ones, and what you can do.
- Identifying the obstacles, barriers, and challenges you face as a mental health leader.
- Guiding you in developing mental health literacy to educate yourself and those across the profession.
- Encouraging the development of future and existing leaders through a realistic mental health leadership model.
- Helping you develop tangible, sustainable, and actionable policy and governance documents that support employees and protect the organisation.
- Structuring a broad mental health program.
- Developing a framework to build a positive culture of safety and wellbeing in your workplace.
- Providing effective support to staff members to prevent them from taking sick leave.
- Providing early support and ensuring a sustainable return to work.

- Lastly, offering a series of templates to help develop a sustainable and accountable mental health and wellbeing program within organisations.

I trust the information in this book has been helpful and will allow you to put everything you've learned into practice.

Thanks for joining me on this journey. All the very best on your personal journey, and good luck!

✧

Annex One

Draft Law Enforcement Policy Statement

Developing A Policy Statement

Commitment to positive mental health benefits everyone in the workplace. It boosts morale, results in lower absenteeism, and increases productivity. It also signifies that an organisation values and respects its workforce, acknowledges the work its employees perform, and supports those dealing with occupational stress and trauma. All employers in first-responder organisations should introduce a written mental health policy statement clearly supporting positive mental health.

Here's a suggested step-by-step process for crafting an effective workplace mental health policy statement:

Step 1 — Review existing health and wellness policies or programs and determine the purpose of your program going forward

If your workplace already has a health or wellness policy, consider updating it to encompass mental health. For assistance, see Supporting Mental Health in First Responders: Recommended Practices.

Step 2 — Draft a statement for your workplace
The policy statement should clearly articulate the organisation's commitment to safeguarding the psychological health, safety, and well-being of its employees and to eliminating the stigma associated with occupational mental health conditions.

Step 3 — Define positive mental health
Explain ways to build resilience, reinforce positive mental health at work, and support those who are struggling with mental health issues.

Step 4 — Apply the policy statement
This should outline the policy's scope. For instance, it applies to permanent, temporary, and contract workers, as well as to interpersonal and electronic communications.

Step 5 — Inform everyone about the policy statement
Ensure all workers, supervisors, and managers are aware of the policy statement through a robust communication strategy. Provide them with copies of it and post the policy statement in visible locations throughout the workplace.

Step 6 — Review the policy statement annually
Include the date the policy becomes effective and the date when the policy statement will be reviewed annually. Develop and revise the organisation's policy statement based on experience and recommended practices. For instance, if a mental health incident has occurred, consider whether there are lessons learned that can be incorporated into your revised policy statement.

Template: Workplace mental health policy statement

Below is an example of a policy statement for law enforcement organisations. It can be adjusted to meet the needs of individual workplaces.

1. Our mental health policy and program
<Organisation Name> is committed to safeguarding the psychological health, safety, and well-being of its employees. We recognise that workplace stress and trauma are health and safety issues that we must address. By establishing a mental health policy and procedures to tackle mental health issues, we can improve the well-being of the organisation and everyone who works for it. We will consistently strive to achieve the highest standards to support positive mental health.

2. Our mental health policy statement
<Organisation Name> fosters a respectful workplace culture free from stigma and compassionate towards anyone who may have a mental health condition. We will incorporate psychological health, safety, and well-being into all aspects of work at all levels throughout the organisation.

3. Positive mental health
We will ensure that leaders are occupationally aware and educated to recognise signs of mental health injury. We will work to raise awareness about mental health issues and foster open dialogue among employees, managers, leadership, and unions. We will confront stigma and make training and support tools available to all workers and employers for their own support and that of their co-workers. This may include access to employee assistance

programmes, peer support, and return-to-work programmes. We will always ensure confidentiality and privacy.

4. Application
This policy applies to all employees of **‹Organisation Name›** in all locations where employees work or attend. It applies in personal dealings and electronic communications.

5. Awareness
This policy applies to all employees of **‹Organisation Name›** in all locations where employees work or are present. It applies in personal dealings and electronic communications.

6. Annual review
This policy statement will be reviewed every year. All workers and managers will receive a copy.

Date created: _____ Annual review date: _____

✧

Annex Two

Draft Law Enforcement Strategic Plan

OUR VISION – Mentally healthy people, mentally healthy communities.

OUR MISSION – To create the best mental health system in the world, characterised by:

- Education
- Accessibility, effectiveness, and efficiency
- Person-led participation
- Policies, services, and programmes that work seamlessly together
- Mental health promotion, prevention, and early intervention

OUR STRATEGIC PRIORITIES for 2022-2025 are to:

- Promote an organisational voice for better mental health
- Highlight the social determinants for mental ill health and advocate for
- enduring changes across the entire organisation
- Deliver value to our staff and the broader mental health ecosystem

We will do this because:
- It is what people want
- It is the optimal way to achieve the system we need — a truly person-led system
- It will enhance the effectiveness of the voice of those with lived experience

We will do this by:
- Building a shared agenda and adopting a collaborative approach
- Partnering with our staff to highlight innovation, influence, and leadership, both within the organisation and among those with lived experience
- At **<Organisation Name>**, we will highlight the social determinants for mental ill health and advocate for authentic and systemic change.

We will do this because:
- It is time to address these systemic issues
- It is necessary to recognise that mental health reform is comprehensive and involves looking beyond the health system

We will do this by:
- Prioritising our policy focus on specific social determinants, based on staff feedback
- Establishing new partnerships across government and related sectors to shift leadership and action beyond health
- Being the 'go to' respected voice on behalf of the mental health system for the related sectors.

✧

Draft Law Enforcement Mental Health Business Case

Project Name

Project Manager

Client

Duration

Executive Summary

- This section should provide a concise version of each of the subsequent sections in your business case.

Mission Statement:

- This section should define the vision, goals, and objectives of the project.

Product/Service:

- This section should explain what the product or service is, and how it fills a niche or meets a need.

Project Definition:

- This section should provide general information about the project, such as an outline of the project plan.

Project Organisation:

- This section should discuss the structure of the project. Is it functional, matrix, projectised, or composite?

Financial Appraisal:

- This section should estimate the cost of executing the project plan over the duration of the project.

Market Assessment:

- This section should research the market opportunities and threats, including competitors.

Marketing Strategy:

- This section should outline how your product or service will be distributed, what its function will be, who the target audience is, etc.

Risk Assessment:

- This section should identify potential risks to your project and formulate strategies to identify and mitigate them.

✧

Annex Four

Draft Law Enforcement Governance Considerations

The 'Mental Health at Work' initiative serves as a comprehensive roadmap for organisations in law enforcement that aspire to encourage, support, and implement exemplary mental health-related programs in the workplace. It is structured around four pillars: People and Wellbeing, Leadership and Commitment, Planning and Risk Management, and Implementation and Evaluation.

People and well-being driver

The People and Wellbeing Driver concentrates on how employees are treated, motivated, supported, and empowered to contribute to the organisation's overall success, as well as to the enhancement of psychological health and safety. This driver emphasises the organisation's efforts to foster and support a respectful and inclusive environment that encourages people to adopt healthy and safe practices in all life aspects and inspires them to continually learn and develop. This focus notably influences the workplace culture within the organisation, especially as the paradigm of the 'workplace' rapidly evolves to hybrid and remote models. As a foundation for establishing a psychologically healthy and safe workplace, people share the responsibility for health, safety, and wellbeing, and treat each other with respect.

Leadership

Leadership is about setting the culture, values, and overall direction for success. It includes demonstrating good governance and meeting the organisation's legal, ethical, and societal obligations. Managing a psychologically healthy and safe workplace is a line-management task, supported either through direct involvement by senior management, or directives from senior leadership. Good leadership is rooted in ethics and values that foster the development and sustainability of psychologically healthy and safe environments.

Planning and risk management

The Planning and Risk Management Driver focuses on developing a Mental Health Plan and establishing measurable goals within the plan. A Mental Health Plan includes a focus on three elements: psychological, physical, and social factors that impact employees' psychological health and safety. All plans, goals, and outcomes are linked to the organisation's Strategic Plan and communicated in a manner that makes the commitment to a psychologically healthy and safe workplace clear to all stakeholders. Planning is based on the identification of workplace psychological health and safety risks and needs. This includes the development of dashboards and measures for leading and lagging indicators. A data-driven health and safety risk management system, founded on continual improvement, is key to achieving desired outcomes and encourages a prevention-based approach to planning.

Implementation and evaluation driver

The Implementation and Evaluation Driver emphasises the selection and design of programs, implementation of activities, and evaluation of integrated mental health and employee wellbeing programs and practices. It includes a disciplined and consistent approach to planning, monitoring, analysing, evaluating, adjusting, and reporting on progress towards desired outcomes. Evaluation focuses on the impact the programs and practices are having on employee psychological health and safety, as well as tangible and intangible benefits, such as value of investment (VOI) and return on investment (ROI).

Key information

Workplace governance helps set expectations across the department. It clearly defines what psychological hazards are and how you will manage them.

Organisations should have a mental health policy, an anti-bullying policy, an anti-discrimination and harassment policy, and a flexible work policy. These demonstrate a commitment to worker wellbeing and a positive workplace culture.

Mental health policy

The aim of a mental health policy is to provide guidance on the responsibilities of both workers and leaders. It should be specific to your workplace.

At a minimum, a workplace mental health policy should include:

- A description of the policy's purpose.
- Details on who is covered by the policy.
- An explanation of what is required by law.

- A clear explanation of psychological hazards, expectations, and behaviour standards (e.g., what is acceptable and unacceptable behaviour).
- References to supporting and/or relevant procedures.
- Details on how complaints or issues are managed and the consequences of not following the policy.
- A process for monitoring and reviewing the policy itself (and the supporting procedures).

Additionally, you should consider:

- Setting specific goals for the policy and aligning it with your organisation's broader objectives.
- Engaging the entire workplace and providing everyone an opportunity to give feedback.
- Ensuring the policy is written in clear and simple English and is tailored to your workers.
- Establishing a robust process to implement the policy and making sure it is accessible to all – be sure to include it in your induction process for new workers.
- Detailing a system to manage, review, and update the policy, for instance, when a law changes.

It is important that departments develop and implement an anti-bullying policy that clearly identifies the expected behaviours and consequences of not complying.

The policy should be developed in consultation with employees and should include:

- A clear statement that the organisation has zero tolerance for workplace bullying in any form and is committed to preventing workplace bullying as part of providing a safe and healthy work environment.

- The expected behaviour standards from everyone in the workplace.
- The procedure for reporting and responding to incidents of workplace bullying.
- The process for managing reports of workplace bullying.

Anti-discrimination and harassment policy

Everyone has the right to work in an environment free of discrimination and harassment and to be treated with dignity and respect.

Having an anti-discrimination and harassment policy can help your team understand what kind of behaviour will and will not be tolerated. The policy should cover:

- Employer and employee rights and responsibilities
- The relevant workplace legislations
- Accepted standards of behaviour
- The consequences for unacceptable conduct
- The process for raising and investigating complaints

Flexible work policy

Providing employees with flexibility in how and where they work can help create a mentally healthy workplace. This could include flexible start and finish times, job sharing, or working from home.

A policy is an excellent way to show that your business supports flexibility and work-life balance. It should include:

- Consultation with employees
- Employee legal rights for requesting flexible work arrangements

- The types of flexible arrangements available in your workplace
- The process for making and responding to flexible work requests
- How agreed flexible arrangements will be monitored and reviewed

Return-to-work program

A return-to-work program is a formal policy outlining procedures for supporting employees to return to the workplace after a physical or psychological work-related injury or illness.

Finally, other elements to consider include:

- Incorporating a mental health component within operational plans
- Infusing a mental health aspect within all risk assessments
- Ensuring all business plans contain tangible references to mental health impacts
- Detailing personal and organisational objectives related to better mental health in individual annual performance management programs

✧

Annex Five

Developing A Business Case

Essential elements of a business case

1. Identify problems and/or opportunities

The aim at this stage is to pinpoint current and emerging problems and opportunities, showcasing the benefits of addressing them. A 'problem' is a cost to be avoided or saved, while an 'opportunity' represents a potential gain. The impact of problems or opportunities should be demonstrated using evidence, including:

- The scale of the problem or opportunity, expressed in monetary terms where possible.
- The timing of the problem or opportunity — when costs and benefits will occur, and how this timeframe influences investment decisions.
- The underlying or root causes of the problem or opportunity.

Key questions to address include:

- Is the problem/opportunity expressed as a clear statement?
- Is the problem/opportunity linked to other problems, programs, and projects?

- How does the problem/opportunity align with relevant government priorities/policy objectives?
- Is the problem/opportunity measured by quantitative and/or qualitative data?
- Has the problem/opportunity been monetised over time?
- What are the assumptions about future trends in drivers (e.g., population, economic growth, technology, climate trends)?
- Have the project/opportunity interrelationships been described?

2. Options analysis

The objective of this stage is to present a wide range of options, including a base case, to address an identified problem or opportunity. You should then assess each of these options through a rigorous process to determine which are likely to benefit the Australian community most. The options analysis should identify a comprehensive list of alternatives to address the problems and opportunities that were identified above.

This list should represent a wide range of reasonable alternatives (both capital and non-capital) and undergo a detailed and evidence-based assessment to determine a shortlist. Consider how individual initiatives and options can be packaged together or better coordinated for a more efficient and effective outcome, and how such options can handle future uncertainty if necessary.

The key deliverables from this stage are:

- A description of each option.
- Anticipated benefit.
- Cost information (including capital expenditure and operating expenditure, where relevant), at a high level.

- A description of the option's expected impact in terms of efficiency, equity, and productivity imposed on or gained by stakeholders by the possible initiatives.

3. Detailed business case development

The purpose of this stage is to refine and finalise your business case by:

- Developing in greater detail the options you shortlisted above to address the problem or opportunity. This includes detail on the costs, benefits, delivery, and risks of each option.
- Refining options based on your analysis. For example, you may refine route alignments, interchanges, or building design standards.
- Ensuring that all factors relevant to the success of an option are comprehensively addressed. For instance, operations, land use planning, and governance structures.

Key questions to address include:

- How was the project contingency estimated?
- For each benefit component, how were the benefits estimated? What are the forecasted benefits?
- What are the characteristics of the underlying demand model?
- Over what timeframe has demand been modelled (month, quarter, year, etc.)?
- Who prepared the capital cost estimates?
- What are the underlying characteristics of the cost-benefit analysis conducted for each project case?
- What are the ongoing costs associated with the project, including maintenance and operating costs?

- Are costs consistent with best practice cost estimation guidelines?
- What sensitivity analysis has been undertaken?
- Are there related initiatives or projects – do the benefits and costs closely relate to, depend upon, or potentially influenced by other initiatives or projects?
- Are there any non-monetised costs and benefits? If so, what are the potential project benefits from them?
- What is the Delivery Strategy and Operations Strategy?
- How will the project be funded and financed?
- What are the unmitigated project risks?
- What is the post-completion review strategy/approach?

Source: https://www.finance.gov.au/government/commonwealth-investment-framework/commonwealth-investments-toolkit/developing-business-case

www.ingramcontent.com/pod-product-compliance
Lightning Source LLC
Chambersburg PA
CBHW052114030426
42335CB00025B/2983